Human Development Network
Health, Nutrition, and Population Series

Addressing HIV/AIDS in East Asia and the Pacific

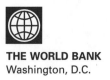

THE WORLD BANK
Washington, D.C.

© 2004 The International Bank for Reconstruction and Development / The World Bank
1818 H Street, NW
Washington, D.C. 20433
Telephone 202-473-1000
Internet www.worldbank.org
E-mail feedback@worldbank.org

1 2 3 4 07 06 05 04

ISBN 0-8213-5916-9
eISBN 0-8213-5917-9

Library of Congress Cataloging-in-Publication Data.

Addressing HIV/AIDS in East Asia and the Pacific.
    p. cm — (Health, nutrition, and population series)
  Includes bibliographical references and index.
  ISBN 0-8213-5916-9
    1. AIDS (Disease)—East Asia. 2. AIDS (Disease)—Pacific Area. 3. World Bank I. World Bank II. Series

  RA643.86.E18A325 2004
  614.5'99392'0095—dc22

2004055291

Addressing HIV/AIDS
in East Asia
and the Pacific

Table of Contents

Foreword   vii

Acknowledgments   ix

Acronyms and Abbreviations   xi

Key Public Health Definitions   xiii

Executive Summary   1
   Characteristics of HIV/AIDS in the East Asia
      and Pacific Region   1
   Lessons from the Region   3
   Partners in the Response: Governments, Donors,
      and Beyond   5
   Five Key Challenges   6
   Strategic Response   7
   World Bank Support: Analytic Work, Funding,
      and Regional Work   9

1 HIV/AIDS in the East Asia and Pacific Region   11
   Characteristics of HIV/AIDS in the EAP Region   11
   The Future of HIV/AIDS in the EAP Region   15
   HIV/AIDS and Beyond: Implications for Other
      Diseases, the Health System, and the Society   16

2 Current National Responses to HIV/AIDS   19
   The Thai Experience: Merging Political Commitment,
      Surveillance, and Civil Society   19

The Cambodian Experience: Using the
   100 Percent Condom Policy 23
The Philippines Experience: A Success Story
   in a Completely Different Context 23
The Indonesian Experience: The Importance
   of Political Commitment in Low-Level Epidemics 24
The Papua New Guinea Experience:
   A Different Epidemic 25
Other Countries Facing Similar Challenges 26

3 Key Challenges 29
Political Commitment and Multisectoral Support 29
Public Health Surveillance and Monitoring
   and Evaluation 30
Prevention 32
Care, Support, and Treatment 34
Strengthening Health Services Delivery 35

4 The World Bank Strategy for HIV/AIDS
   in the East Asia and Pacific Region 37
Lessons from the World Bank over the Last Decade 37
Strategic Directions 41
Analytic and Advisory Work 45
Lending and Funding for HIV/AIDS in the EAP Region 45
Regional Activities 46

Conclusion 47

Annex 1 Classification of the Epidemic 49
Annex 2 Country Overviews 51
Annex 3 Snapshot of Estimated Number and
   Risk Behaviors of Injecting Drug Users
   and Commercial Sex Workers in the EAP Region 65
Annex 4 Infectious Disease Epidemiology 71
Annex 5 Epidemiological Projections of HIV/AIDS
   in East Asia 75
Annex 6 Tuberculosis 79
Annex 7 Overview of Current Blood Safety Policy Status 81
Annex 8 Approved HIV-Related Projects Under
   the Global Fund for EAP Region 85

Notes 87

References 91

Bibliography 95

Web Sites 97

Index 99

Foreword

Combating the spread of HIV/AIDS presents the international community with one of its most difficult global challenges. The tragedy now unfolding in Sub-Saharan Africa does not reflect the extent of the disease's devastating effects on populations around the world, and there is now growing concern that the countries of the East Asia and Pacific Region may share a similar fate unless timely and appropriate measures can be taken.

This strategy note is intended to help chart the nature of the epidemic in the East Asia and Pacific Region; to survey some of the successful practices being pioneered in its cities, provinces, and countries; and to offer suggestions as to how the distinct characteristics of the HIV/AIDS epidemic faced in each country can be addressed by effective and comprehensive responses.

This regional strategy recognizes that the challenge posed by HIV/AIDS is further complicated by changing social patterns, weak health systems, high rates of tuberculosis, and large populations engaged in high-risk behaviors. Within this context, responses must take into account five key challenges: political commitment and multisectoral support; public health surveillance and monitoring and evaluation; prevention; care, support, and treatment; and health services delivery.

The sheer scale of the HIV/AIDS epidemic will require ongoing, dynamic cooperation among a broad coalition of stakeholders. It is hoped that this strategy—drawn from the World Bank's experience as well as that of the many partners with whom the Bank is working—will help inform future discussion and action.

Jemal-ud-din Kassum
Vice President
East Asia and Pacific Region

Acknowledgments

This strategy note was prepared by Michael Borowitz, Elizabeth Wiley, Fadia Saadah, and Enis Baris. Significant inputs were sought and provided by EASHD staff. The strategy note was received, reviewed, and endorsed by Emmanuel Jimenez, EASHD Director. Enis Baris prepared the initial concept and commissioned most of the work on which the strategy was built. In addition, special thanks to Debrework Zewdie and Susan Stout for their help and support in preparing the manuscript and to Olusoji Adeyi, Martha Ainsworth, Gisele Biyoo, Donald Bundy, Dave Burrows, Sungwook Ryan Chung, Nick Crofts, Eric de Roodenbeke, Phoebe Folger, Peter Heywood, Janet Hohnen, Silvia Holschneider, Dale Huntington, Samuel Lieberman, Tony Lisle, Joan MacNeil, Elizabeth Mziray, Son Nam Nguyen, Elizabeth Pisani, Alex Preker, Alex Ross, Swarup Sarkar, Jagadish Upadhyay, Neff Walker, Shiyong Wang, Diana Weil, David Wilson, and Abdo Yazbek. Some of the background work was provided by a number of consultants, including Julian Gold, Alex Wilson, Don Smith, Elizabeth Dax, Vivian Lin, Alison Heywood, James Chin, and Sumera Haque. The authors also thank their colleagues in partner agencies, especially UNAIDS, WHO, USAID, JICA, AusAID, DFID, GFATM, and ADB. The text was edited by Meta de Coquereaumont, with Bruce Ross-Larson and Elizabeth McCrocklin, at Communications Development Incorporated.

The authors of this strategy note are grateful to the World Bank for having published the strategy as an HNP Discussion Paper. The preparation of this regional strategy was cofinanced by the Global HIV/AIDS Program of the World Bank through the UNAIDS Unified Budget and Workplan (UBW) and by the East Asia and Pacific Region of the World Bank.

Acronyms and Abbreviations

ADB	Asian Development Bank
AIDS	Acquired immune deficiency syndrome
ASEAN	Association of Southeast Asian Nations
ART	Antiretroviral treatment
AusAID	The Australian government's overseas aid program
CAS	Country assistance strategy
CDC	Centers for Disease Control and Prevention (United States)
CSW	Commercial sex worker
DFID	Department for International Development (United Kingdom)
DOTS	Directly observed treatment, short course
EAP	East Asia and Pacific
EFA	Education for All
FSW	Female sex worker
GFATM	Global Fund to Fight AIDS, Tuberculosis, and Malaria
HIV	Human immunodeficiency virus
IDU	Injecting drug user
MOH	Ministry of Health
NGO	Nongovernmental organization
OECD	Organisation for Economic Co-operation and Development
STI	Sexually transmitted infection
TB	Tuberculosis
UN	United Nations

UNAIDS	Joint United Nations Programme on HIV/AIDS
UNESCO	United Nations Educational, Scientific, and Cultural Organization
USAID	United States Agency for International Development
VCT	Voluntary counseling and testing
WHO	World Health Organization

Key Public Health Definitions

Antiretrovirals: Drugs that inhibit the replication of HIV—generally three drugs in combination—and thus extend life expectancy.

Behavioral surveillance: Tracking trends in behavior over time that carry a risk for HIV infection, such as sharing needles or having unprotected sex with multiple partners.

Epidemic: The occurrence in a community or region of an illness or group of illnesses of similar nature, clearly in excess of normal expectancy or in excess of the endemic level.

Incidence rate: The number of new cases of a disease over a defined period of time, generally a year, divided by the population at risk of acquiring the disease during the same period of time.

Opportunistic infections: As HIV infection decreases human immunity, individuals are more susceptible to other infectious diseases, which are often the proximate cause of death.

Pandemic: A disease epidemic across a wide area, usually crossing international boundaries and affecting a large number of people.

Prevalence rate: The total number of cases of disease at a certain time divided by the population at risk of having the disease.

Reproductive rate: The average number of new infections caused by one infected individual in a native population. If the rate is greater than one, a self-sustaining epidemic is possible; if it is less than one, the infection becomes extinct.

Sentinel HIV surveillance: Measuring trends over time in the prevalence of HIV in defined populations with different levels of risk behavior. These populations include those with high-risk behavior such as commercial sex workers, injecting drug users, and men who have sex with men. They may also include populations more representative of the general population, such as pregnant women, prisoners, and others, depending on the culture.

Addressing HIV/AIDS in East Asia and the Pacific

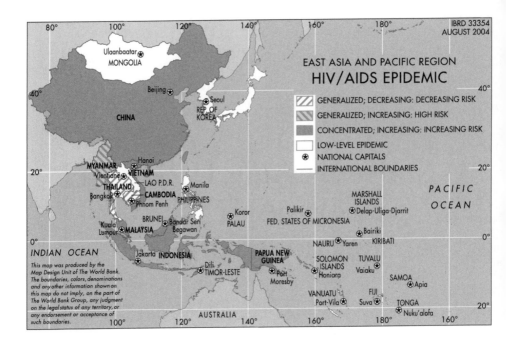

Executive Summary

With almost half the world's population, Asia will determine the future of the global human immunodeficiency virus/acquired immune deficiency syndrome (HIV/AIDS) pandemic. If prevalence rates in China, Indonesia, and India increase to numbers similar to those seen in Thailand and Cambodia, the rate of HIV/AIDS would double globally. Such growth would be devastating for individuals—and for the region's health systems, economies, and social fabric. HIV/AIDS is therefore a multisectoral development challenge and, consequently, a corporate priority for the World Bank.

This report outlines a strategic direction for the World Bank in its multisectoral response to HIV/AIDS in the East Asia and Pacific (EAP) Region. It describes the risk of a large-scale HIV/AIDS epidemic in the region. It also spells out what can be done to avert the growth of HIV/AIDS—and what government, civil society, and other partners are doing. And it identifies how the World Bank can assist at the country and regional levels. The World Bank will work with countries, civil society, the private sector, donors, and other key players to formulate country-specific strategies that try to respond to the needs of the population.

Characteristics of HIV/AIDS in the East Asia and Pacific Region

In trying to predict the course of the epidemic in East Asia, preconceived notions of the trajectory of HIV/AIDS in other parts of the world may not be applicable. East Asia is likely to experience concentrated epidemics among groups that practice high-risk behaviors, with spread to their part-

1

ners and their children. This could lead to large epidemics, because a relatively high percentage of the population engages in high-risk behaviors.

The Joint United Nations Programme on HIV/AIDS (UNAIDS) predicts a staggering 11 million new cases of HIV/AIDS in the region by 2010. However, this projection is based on limited data. Before accurate projections can be developed, more needs to be known about the number of people who are affected by the disease and the number of people who practice behaviors that put them at risk.

In the EAP Region, the epidemic generally begins at a low level among commercial sex workers regularly having unprotected sex with clients, injecting drug users sharing needles and syringes, or men having unprotected sex with men. As HIV spreads among them, it becomes more heavily concentrated in these populations. It could then spread among these (often overlapping) populations—and possibly to the general population.[1] When HIV comes close to saturation in populations with high-risk behaviors and HIV rates grow to greater than 1 percent among the general population, the epidemic is considered to be generalized. The trajectory of growth depends on the size of the at-risk populations and their overlaps, but there is significant potential for growth. In this region, the data suggest that countries are categorized[2] as:

- **Generalized:** Thailand, Cambodia, Myanmar.

- **Concentrated:** Papua New Guinea, China, Indonesia, Vietnam, Malaysia.

- **Low level:** Mongolia, Lao People's Democratic Republic, the Philippines, Timor Leste, Pacific Island Member States.[3]

The preceding list is based on the 2002 UNAIDS data. Other sources of information may lead to a slightly different classification.

Because AIDS makes people more susceptible to opportunistic infections, it would trigger concomitant growth in tuberculosis (TB) in the region, which already accounts for almost a third of the global TB burden. Given these extremely high rates of TB, increases in HIV would lead to a dangerous dual epidemic. Globally, tuberculosis has already become the leading cause of death among people with HIV, accounting for about a third of the AIDS deaths worldwide (UNAIDS 2000).

Increases in HIV/AIDS and tuberculosis would boost demand for health services and put added stress on already overburdened public health systems, particularly in providing services to the poor. The effects would extend beyond the health sector, as families would lose wage-earners and spend their limited resources on medical care. HIV/AIDS could also disrupt the social fabric by breaking up families, creating orphans, and forcing more households into poverty. In general, HIV/AIDS could lead to a significant reduction in human capital, by taking the lives of youths, and to slower economic growth. HIV/AIDS is thus a threat to development and to reaching the Millennium Development Goals.

Lessons from the Region

In a region as diverse as EAP, there are many lessons that can be learned. Some highlights of the fight against HIV/AIDS in various contexts include experiences from Thailand, the Philippines, Indonesia, and Papua New Guinea.

In the face of a major epidemic, Thailand led the way in prevention programs, mobilizing civil society and building political commitment. By 1992, 31 percent of commercial sex workers were HIV-positive, and there were signs of HIV spreading to the heterosexual population. The national response was strong, swift, and comprehensive, thanks to strong political commitment from the king and prime minister. This multisectoral response was complemented by a sophisticated system of surveillance, including serological surveillance of the general population, sentinel surveillance of groups practicing high-risk behaviors, and behavioral surveillance monitoring risky behavior. This information was backed by strong leadership to support HIV prevention programs among commercial sex workers and their clients. The result: a profound decline in high-risk behavior, which reduced new cases of HIV and eventually decreased the level of HIV in the population.

But HIV/AIDS transmission remains high among injecting drug users in Thailand, and prevention programs have been cut back, particularly since the Asian economic crisis in 1998. There is some concern that the behavior changes early in the epidemic could diminish as the perceived risks decline and prevention programs reach fewer people.

The Philippines provides another success story for the region but in a completely different context. The epidemic in the Philippines has been stemmed by a set of contextual factors: differing commercial sexual practices, low rates of injecting drug use, high rates of circumcision, and fewer ulcerative sexually transmitted infections. The country's measured response to the epidemic, including national law reform to reduce the likelihood of discrimination, widely available voluntary counseling and testing services, and a fair sentinel surveillance system, has helped to keep the prevalence low and stable.

Indonesia points to the need to maintain political commitment to prevention in the low-level stage of the epidemic. In 1996 the government recognized the importance of an early intervention to prevent an epidemic and mobilized initiatives and funding. Several programs were designed to respond to the projected epidemic, including a World Bank-funded project that became effective in 1996. However, many of the efforts were not sustained or scaled up. For example, the World Bank project was closed in 1999 without implementing many of its planned activities. Several factors played into this, including the severe economic crisis and limited capacity. Responsibility for HIV/AIDS was split into several parts of the Ministry of Health, and there was limited coordination. Capacity among nongovernmental organizations for preventive activities and support from some sectors of civil society, particularly religious groups, was also limited.

Even so, HIV prevalence remained low, and the predicted epidemic did not materialize. But the trajectory of HIV/AIDS in Indonesia has since changed, with HIV prevalence rates of more than 60 percent among injecting drug users in some areas of the country. Recently, government commitment appears to be increasing, and a new HIV/AIDS strategy embraces HIV prevention for groups that practice high-risk behaviors.

Limited capacity and cultural mores different from other countries in the region place Papua New Guinea at risk for an epidemic similar to those in Sub-Saharan Africa. Despite numerous alerts raised in the early 1990s to the emerging epidemic, few persons in positions of leadership acknowledged HIV/AIDS as an issue of concern. After recognition of the problem, however, early efforts became difficult to sustain. The National AIDS Committee functioned only sporadically from 1988 to 1994, and efforts in the early 1990s to establish a sentinel surveillance system faltered. More recent efforts have revitalized some programming; however, to date, limited capacity in the health system, poor implementation of HIV programs in general, and a lack of human resources have hampered efforts. In addition, the breakdown of traditional methods of social control in Papua New Guinea, combined with the cash economy, urbanization, and greater mobility, has resulted in significant changes in sexual behavior. These factors place Papua New Guinea at risk for developing a large, heterosexual HIV/AIDS epidemic.

Other countries will face similar challenges. It would be a difficult task to define the depth and breadth of lessons learned in all countries throughout the region. The examples given, however, show the broad range of experiences and highlight some important lessons. The concentrated epidemics of China, Vietnam, and Malaysia also exhibit a mixed fare of projects, responses, and inputs. Unfortunately there is strong potential for HIV/AIDS growth in these countries, particularly China.

China's emerging epidemic is considered to be the next big challenge on the horizon. HIV and AIDS cases are increasing, and there is spread from high-risk populations to the general population (China MOH/UNAIDS 2003). China has made dramatic progress in moving toward a system of voluntary blood donations and creating the infrastructure necessary to ensure the safety of the blood supply. In addition, the Chinese central government recently reaffirmed its commitment to achieving the goals of the United Nations General Assembly Special Session on HIV/AIDS (UNGASS). The government plans to improve laws and regulations, to launch public awareness campaigns, to protect the rights of people living with HIV/AIDS, to increase international cooperation on HIV/AIDS, and to provide antiretrovirals. Many other countries have created similar national AIDS strategies, but actions are now needed. The way these and other strategies and lessons are adopted and adapted within the region will determine the future of the epidemic and the social and economic landscape of Asian society.

Partners in the Response: Governments, Donors, and Beyond

Strong political commitment is a key element in confronting the epidemic; however, resources are also important. Although there has been a high level of commitment from many governments, funding has been low. The main source of funding for HIV/AIDS prevention and surveillance in the region has come from development agencies working alongside governments. The main development partners have been the World Bank; the Asian Development Bank; the U.N. agencies (especially UNAIDS); the large bilateral development agencies; the Global Fund to Fight AIDS, Tuberculosis, and Malaria; and the World Health Organization. Nongovernmental organizations are also offering key services and information.

Although cumulative lending in the region for HIV/AIDS stands at more than $100 million, making the World Bank an important financier of HIV/AIDS projects in the region, the structure of those in the fight against HIV/AIDS has been changing rapidly, which will have an impact on World

Bank funding. The Global Fund channels a large amount of resources to countries that often lack full capacity to implement or support programs. However, it is largely a funding agency and is not designed to assist with the implementation of programs. As a result, new demands are being placed on governments and donors. Implementation and technical assistance will have to be provided by other agencies, for example, bilaterals, the World Bank, and other donors.

This changing landscape makes it difficult to predict the exact role that the World Bank will play in the region, especially in relation to demand for World Bank lending/grants for HIV/AIDS. However, even in an era of increased grant funding through the Global Fund and other bilaterals, the World Bank may play an important role in resource mobilization for HIV/AIDS. Demand for analytic and advisory services and capacity-building efforts is also likely to increase. In addition, the Bank will continue its role as a co-convenor of multiple sectors, its long-term presence in countries, and its multisectoral programs.

Five Key Challenges

The EAP Region could avert a large HIV/AIDS epidemic if countries introduce effective HIV/AIDS programs that address five key challenges:

- *Political commitment and multisectoral support.* Given the sensitivity of the disease, political commitment is key to effective HIV/AIDS programs. Preventing HIV among socially marginalized groups requires a multisectoral response, particularly an enabling legal environment with the support of law enforcement.

- *Public health surveillance, monitoring, and evaluation.* Knowledge of the exact numbers of those with HIV and those practicing high-risk behaviors is extremely limited. More information is essential to estimate the potential growth of the epidemic and to allocate resources and efforts accordingly.

- *Prevention.* Prevention has been shown to be a cost-effective method of abating the epidemic. There is a wide scope for improving HIV prevention, particularly among groups that practice high-risk behaviors (commercial sex workers, injecting drug users, men who have sex with men, and migrant workers).

- *Care, support, and treatment.* Demand is growing throughout the region for antiretroviral therapy. Treatment must also include care and support—including psychosocial support, voluntary counseling and testing, and care for the dying.

- *Health services delivery.* Prevention, care, support, and treatment have to be delivered by public health and social care systems, alongside the private sector, including nongovernmental organizations. There is a definite need to strengthen and build capacity to respond to the emerging needs of the epidemic.

Strategic Response

The World Bank strategy will respond to these challenges by developing country-specific strategies based on the needs of the country and the stage of the epidemic in the country. These HIV/AIDS country strategy notes will be the basis for World Bank engagement. They will be designed in concert with national strategic HIV/AIDS plans created by governments and the World Bank Country Assistance Strategies. The HIV/AIDS strategy notes will provide specific work plans that incorporate some mix of the following tools: analytic and advisory work, lending, and regional activities. They will be designed to be flexible and innovative, focusing on the five key challenges.

Political Commitment and Multisectoral Support

An important part of making progress in any HIV/AIDS program is the use of communications to build the political understanding and commitment across a broad spectrum of sectors (for example, health, education, transport, and so forth) and to increase public awareness and support for HIV/AIDS prevention programs within countries. Analytic work and lending (granting) operations will help identify key stakeholders, their relative importance, and their institutional setting. These tools will also assist in identifying the key sectors and help the World Bank do a better job of integrating multisectoral approaches in country work.

Public Health Surveillance, Monitoring, and Evaluation

Public health surveillance. Good estimates of the number of injecting drug users and the number of commercial sex workers and the percentage of the population visiting them do not exist in most countries. To estimate the growth of the epidemic, one needs to know the size of populations at risk and the overlaps among groups practicing high-risk behavior. This information is rarely known because it is governed by complex social taboos, with the behavior sometimes illegal and the population hidden. Thus it is necessary to use several methods to obtain this information, including routine information systems, surveys, and qualitative research. More funding is required for regular behavioral surveillance and social science research on sexual and drug-using behaviors and for increasing the capacity to conduct this research in local universities and government agencies.

Monitoring and evaluation. A key objective is to assist countries in monitoring and evaluating the effectiveness of HIV/AIDS programs. One element of this work will be policy dialogue with governments on spending on surveillance and prevention among groups that practice high-risk behavior through the development of National Health Accounts for HIV/AIDS. The World Bank will also work with governments to develop and implement monitoring and evaluation systems, including coverage of interventions for prevention and care, support, and treatment. In addition, the World Bank is assisting countries in developing approaches for monitoring and evaluation systems at the local level through the Global HIV/AIDS Monitoring and Evaluation Support Team.[4]

Prevention

Although prevention programs exist among groups with high-risk behaviors, they are often small pilot projects. It is important to work with governments to understand the scale needed for prevention programs to have an epidemiological impact. It is also important to understand sexual and drug-using networks and their overlap to gain more knowledge concerning the potential growth of the epidemic and to learn how to intervene effectively. There is a risk that, over time, prevention programs will receive less attention. It is essential to maintain and strengthen these interventions as a key pillar of the fight against AIDS.

Care, Support, and Treatment

Analytic work is needed to understand how to operationalize issues related to antiretroviral therapy in the context of relatively weak systems of service delivery, including the private sector. Furthermore, antiretroviral therapy needs to be embedded into a large system of care and support, including social services and care for the dying.

Health Services Delivery

The World Bank will work with governments to help in the formulation of better policies for both the public and the private sectors to improve access to care, support, and treatment. This will mean that the growing demand for treatment with antiretroviral therapy, now being met in the private sector, will need to be addressed. In addition, strengthening the coordination between TB and HIV/AIDS programs to ensure maximum effectiveness and efficiency is important. Finally, overall strengthening of the health care system and of absorptive capacity within the broader government is key for delivery of HIV/AIDS interventions.

World Bank Support: Analytic Work, Funding, and Regional Work

Analytic work in the region will focus on gathering and sharing knowledge in relation to the five key challenges. This will include both country-specific and regional pieces. World Bank lending (granting) will need to be guided by the specific country assistance strategies and needs. The Bank will also work toward strengthening the collaboration with other sectors and mainstreaming HIV/AIDS into other lending projects, such as those for infrastructure and education. A broad set of lending instruments and options for client countries to address the multisectoral nature of the disease and the diverse needs across the region is available. Another area in which there could be added value is the development of regional tools that can be utilized by several countries in coordination with other partners. These could include analytic work, knowledge-sharing initiatives, and other similar programs. In disseminating lessons, the EAP Region will work closely with the World Bank Institute to strengthen and build institutional capacity for controlling HIV/AIDS throughout the region.

Working together with governments, civil society, and other development partners, the World Bank can play a critical role in addressing the risks associated with concentrated HIV/AIDS epidemics in the EAP Region to prevent the region from becoming the future epicenter of HIV/AIDS.

CHAPTER 1

HIV/AIDS
in the East Asia and
Pacific Region

The East Asia and Pacific (EAP) Region of the World Bank is the world's most populous region. In such a large and diverse area, the HIV/AIDS epidemic is as varied as the countries involved—from 12 fishermen with HIV in Tuvalu, with potentially devastating consequences for the country's fishing-based economy, to an estimated 1 million people infected in China by the end of 2002 with profound implications for the health system. As a region, EAP has an estimated 2.3 million adults and children living with HIV/AIDS, of the global burden of 42 million (Gold and Wilson 2002).

Characteristics of HIV/AIDS in the EAP Region

A sense of the magnitude of the HIV/AIDS epidemic can be drawn from a rough classification based on prevalence rates, which represent the total number of people with the disease as a share of the population at risk (Table 1 and Annex 1). It should be noted, however, that there are numerous discrepancies in HIV/AIDS data. To ensure a minimal level of standardization, numbers in Table 1 were first taken from 2002 UNAIDS data when possible. Other sources of information may lead to a slightly different classification (for example, Papua New Guinea may be classified as a generalized epidemic based on recent national surveillance).

- **Generalized:** Cambodia, Thailand, and Myanmar. HIV is close to saturation in populations whose members practice high-risk behaviors, and

11

Table 1 Overview of HIV/AIDS Epidemic in EAP, 2001 (unless otherwise indicated)

Country	Adult (ages 15–49) Prevalence rate (percent)	Population (adult population, ages 15–49) (million)	Est. number living with HIV/AIDS (est. number of adults living with HIV/AIDS)	HIV prevalence, selected populations, major urban areas (percent)					GNI per capita 2000 (US$)
				Female commercial sex workers	Injecting drug users	Male patients with sexually transmitted infections	Women in antenatal care clinics[a]	Women in antenatal care clinics outside major urban areas	
Generalized									
Cambodia	2.7	13.4 (6.3)	170,000 (160,000)	26.3–31 (2000/2001)	—	8.5 (1994)	2.7 (2000)	0.6–5.7 (2000)	270
Myanmar	—[b]	48.3 (25.8)	180,000– 400,000	26.0–50.0 (2000)	37.1–63 (2000)	12.1–13.0 (2000)	2.0–3.5 (2000)	0.0–5.3 (2000)	390
Thailand	1.8	63.6 (36.6)	670,000 (650,000)	6.7–10.5 (2000)	39.6–50 (2000)	2.5 (2000)	1.6–1.6 (2000)	0.4–5.3 (2000)	2,020
Concentrated									
China	0.1	1,284.9 (726)	850,000 (850,000)	0.0–10.3 (2000)	0.0–80 (2000)	0.0–1.3 (2000)	0.0 (2000)	0.5 (2000)	840
Indonesia	0.1	214.8 (118)	120,000 (120,000)	Up to 2.0–27 (2002)	19–48 (2001/2002)	—	0.0 (1999)	0.0 (1996)	580
Malaysia	0.4	22.6 (11.8)	42,000 (41,000)	2.05–6.3 (1996)	16.8 (1996)	4.2 (1996)	—	0.0–0.7 (1996)	3,250
Papua New Guinea	0.7	4.9 (2.4)	17,000 (16,000)	16.0 (2002)	—	7.0 (1998)	0.2 (1995)	0.0 (1992)	670
Vietnam	0.3	79 (43.3)	130,000 (130,000)	4.2–6.0 (2002/2003)	26.8–30.4 (2003)	2.0–3.2 (2002/2003)	0.4 (2003)	0.0–0.3 (1999)	390

Low level

Lao PDR	<0.1	5.4 (2.5)	1,400 (1,300)	1.0 (2000)	2.0	0.0 (1998)	—	290
Mongolia	<0.1	2.5 (1.4)	<100 (<100)	—	No reported cases	0.0 (1989)	—	390
Philippines	<0.1	77 (39.6)	9,400 (9,400)	0.3 (1994)	1.0	0.0 (1994)	—	1,020

Blank cells: Information not available.

Note: There are numerous discrepancies in data on HIV. Therefore, to ensure a minimal level of standardization, numbers were first taken from UNAIDS when possible. See Annex 2 for more data. Not all countries in the EAP Region are listed. These are the primary countries that will be targeted for World Bank HIV/AIDS programming or are countries of concern because prevalence rates are either high or expected to be high in the near future.

a. Antenatal care is not always indicative of prevalence in the general population (as in Indonesia, where it is not a part of regular sentinel surveillance).

b. In Myanmar, UNAIDS does not report prevalence, but it does report the estimated number of HIV cases. This gives an estimate of prevalence ranging from 0.7 to 1.54.

Source: *Epidemiological Fact Sheets by Country–2002 Updates* (UNAIDS/WHO 2002); *Report on the Global HIV/AIDS Epidemic 2002* (UNAIDS 2002); *HIV/AIDS in Asia and the Pacific Region* (WHO 2001); *World Development Indicators 2001* (World Bank 2001) (http://www.worldbank.org/data/wdi2001/); Burrows 2003, Personal communication, The Burnet Institute, Melbourne, Australia; Khorloo 2003; Reid and Costigan 2002; Feng, undated; NASB/MOH 2003; NASB 2002; World Bank, 2003; Pisani and others 2003.

HIV rates are greater than 1 percent among the general population, as measured by antenatal clinic attendees.

- **Concentrated:** China, Indonesia, Malaysia, Papua New Guinea, and Vietnam. HIV prevalence surpasses 5 percent in one or more subpopulations presumed to practice high-risk behavior, as measured by sentinel surveillance of groups such as commercial sex workers and injecting drug users, but prevalence among the general population is less than 1 percent.

- **Low level:** Lao PDR, Mongolia, Pacific Island Member States, the Philippines, and Timor Leste. HIV prevalence is less than 5 percent in all known subpopulations presumed to practice high-risk behavior.

Cambodia has the highest prevalence, with an estimated 2.7 percent of the adult population living with HIV/AIDS. Myanmar is presumed to have a generalized epidemic, with an estimated 180,000–400,000 adults living with HIV, or prevalence between 0.70 and 1.54 percent. Thailand is next, with an estimated prevalence rate among adults of 1.8 percent.

Although this typology is useful, it paints with a very broad brush. As this classification system looks only at the national level, it can mask regional or local prevalence rates or patterns (FHI/USAID 2001a). In EAP, with huge countries like China, this is an important distinction. So this classification serves only as a broad categorization, best used with country and region-specific analysis.

The prevalence rate does not tell the whole story.[5] One also needs to know the number of new infections (incidence) to understand the epidemic's direction. Other keys to the severity of the epidemic are the size of the population whose members practice risk behaviors and the nature of the behaviors. The main factor driving Asian epidemics is the high percentage of the population in groups engaging in risky behavior (commercial sex workers, injecting drug users) and the overlap among these groups. Many countries in the region have a large number of commercial sex workers, visited by a significant percentage of the male population. There are increasing numbers of injecting drug users, and some resort to commercial sex to fund their addiction (see Annex 3). The number and behaviors of men having sex with men also plays a role. But without better knowledge of these groups, it is hard to fully understand the epidemic. (More information on the epidemiology of HIV/AIDS is available in Annex 4.)

Regional integration can also facilitate the spread of HIV/AIDS. Though linkages between HIV/AIDS and migration and mobility are complex, they are evident in many parts of the world. The most obvious factor is labor migration, with vast numbers of people traveling between and within countries. Of the Filipinos reported to be living with HIV, 28 percent are workers who have returned home after working abroad (UNAIDS 2002). There are also regional networks trafficking in women and illicit drugs. These regional factors create the preconditions of high-risk behavior—behavior that can ignite an HIV/AIDS epidemic. Programs to mitigate the risks of mobility must address all stages of migration with a regional approach extending beyond country borders.

The Future of HIV/AIDS in the EAP Region

Although there are limited data, predictions about the epidemic in EAP range from rates similar to those in Sub-Saharan Africa to estimates of less than 1 percent prevalence in the general population (Annex 5).

Three Predictions

- *High-range predictions: EAP as the epicenter of the epidemic.* The predictions of large-scale growth of Asian epidemics are based on the experience of Sub-Saharan Africa, where concentrated epidemics began in groups practicing high-risk behavior, and then HIV spread to the general population. Under this scenario, Asia is at great risk of becoming the epicenter of the HIV/AIDS epidemic in the next decade (Eberstadt 2002).

- *Low-range predictions: HIV/AIDS may not be a large problem in Asia.* In contrast, low-range estimates predict Asian HIV/AIDS epidemics are constrained by low-risk sexual behavior in the general population (Chin 2003). Some analysts believe that the Asian HIV/AIDS epidemics will never become the generalized epidemics that are ravaging Sub-Saharan Africa. Multiple, overlapping partners and high rates of sexually transmitted diseases, which drive the Sub-Saharan African epidemics, do not exist in the region. Since risky behavior in the general population is low in Asia, HIV/AIDS will stay in concentrated pockets and will not spread widely through the general, heterosexual population.

- *Mid-range predictions: High-risk behavior drives a moderate epidemic.* The U.S. Agency for International Development (USAID) commissioned a consortium led by Tim Brown and Wiwat Peerapatinapokin to develop a dynamic model of HIV/AIDS transmission to understand the trajectory of HIV/AIDS in Thailand. The Asian Epidemic Model was used in Thailand and Cambodia where behavioral data were available and predicted that growth of the epidemic would not be constrained by low-risk behavior in the general population. The growth is driven by the high rate of high-risk behavior in the population, with reports of over 25 percent of men having sex outside of long-term partnerships.

Difficult to Tell Precise Extent of Epidemic: Call for Action

Although the estimates for HIV/AIDS in the region vary widely, there is no doubt of the strong potential for the epidemic to grow in many countries, such as China, Indonesia, and Papua New Guinea. In the EAP Region, there are no large generalized epidemics with prevalence greater than 5 percent with growth sustained by heterosexual transmission in the general population.[6] The main characteristic of Asian epidemics is they are *concentrated* epidemics in large populations of people practicing high-risk behaviors, with some spread to the general population. Even the generalized epidemics of Cambodia, Myanmar, and Thailand are primarily large, concentrated epidemics. However, the Joint United Nations Programme on HIV/AIDS (UNAIDS) estimates suggest that epidemics can be sizable without HIV/AIDS becoming a generalized epidemic in the entire population. It has been estimated that significant epidemics beyond 3–5 percent prevalence could occur in the adult population simply because of the size of the groups that practice high-risk behavior. (Cambodia Working Group on HIV/AIDS Projection 2002; Thai Working Group on HIV/AIDS Projections 2001). And because many of these groups overlap, the epidemic can become self-sustaining even without generalizing to low-risk populations. It is estimated that even without a generalized epidemic in the adult population, large epidemics of grave public health concern could occur, leading to an additional 11 million infections in the EAP Region by 2010[7] (Figure 1).

HIV/AIDS and Beyond: Implications for Other Diseases, the Health System, and the Society

HIV/AIDS has significant effects beyond the number of people infected with HIV/AIDS. Many people who develop AIDS may also develop a number of other opportunistic infections. HIV/AIDS lowers immunity and makes people more susceptible to infectious diseases such as tuberculosis,

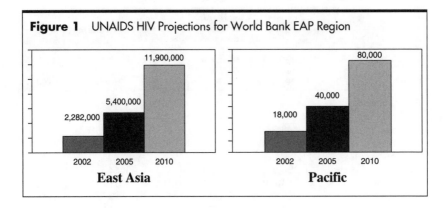

Figure 1 UNAIDS HIV Projections for World Bank EAP Region

already a significant challenge in many of the EAP countries. All countries in EAP have tuberculosis rates greater than 100 cases per 100,000, which is significantly high (Table 2 and Annex 6). Of the 22 countries identified by the WHO as bearing the highest burden of tuberculosis, seven are in EAP (Box 1). HIV/AIDS also makes tuberculosis and other infectious diseases more difficult to control by straining health systems.

As HIV/AIDS epidemics mature, as in Thailand, and the number of people living with HIV/AIDS rises, so does the need for access to care, including antiretroviral therapy and scarce hospital resources. However, the effects extend beyond the health care system. A large-scale HIV/AIDS epidemic also threatens development by slowing the growth of human capital—and ultimately economic growth. Within this larger context of deteriorating human capital is an increasingly vulnerable population of children affected by HIV/AIDS. UNAIDS estimates that globally children orphaned by AIDS now number 14.0 million (UNAIDS 2002). HIV/AIDS not only leaves children without families, it also strains education systems, weakening demand, eroding quality, widening the gender gap, and increasing sector costs (World Bank 2002). If the epidemic grows in EAP, the rising numbers of AIDS orphans will have a lasting effect on the region. In addition, young women are especially vulnerable to HIV/AIDS. This and other gender dimensions of the epidemic must also be addressed.

The good news, however, is that the HIV/AIDS epidemic can be controlled. The following chapters review countries' responses to HIV/AIDS, identify progress made, and define the key challenges that must be confronted to halt the growth of the epidemic in Asia.

Table 2 Estimated Number of Individuals with Tuberculosis

Country	Population (thousands, 2001)	Estimated number of adults and children living with HIV/AIDS (2001)	Adult prevalence rate of HIV (percent, 2001)	Estimated cases of tuberculosis (2003)	
				Number	Rate per 100,000
Generalized					
Cambodia[a]	13,441	170,000	2.7	78,564	585
Myanmar[a]	48,364	—	—	78,473	162
Thailand[a]	63,584	670,000	1.8	85,870	135
Concentrated					
China[a]	1,284,972	850,000	0.1	1,447,948	113
Indonesia[a]	214,840	120,000	0.1	581,847	271
Malaysia	22,633	42,000	0.4	27,119	120
Papua New Guinea	4,920	17,000	0.7	11,602	236
Vietnam[a]	79,175	130,000	0.3	141,353	179
Low level					
Timor-Leste	—	—	—	—	—
Lao PDR	5,403	1,400	<0.1	8,512	158
Mongolia	2,559	<100	<0.1	4,969	194
Philippines[a]	77,131	9,400	<0.1	228,931	297

Blank cells: Information not available.
[a] Part of the WHO highest burden countries responsible for 80 percent of global tuberculosis.
Source: Epidemiological Fact Sheets by Country–2002 Updates (UNAIDS/WHO 2002) (AIDS data); *WHO Report 2003: Global Tuberculosis Control: Surveillance, Planning, Financing* (WHO 2003) (tuberculosis data).

Box 1 Tuberculosis in China: A Growing Threat

As one of the 22 countries highlighted by the World Health Organization (WHO) as accounting for 80 percent of the global burden of tuberculosis, China has the second highest number of cases, though they have decreased significantly since China introduced DOTS (Directly Observed Therapy, Short-Course) as part of its national tuberculosis control program. The World Bank has been a key development partner in providing support for the pilot implementation of DOTS in 13 provinces (efforts in 10 other provinces were funded by the government). This was followed by a successor project in 2002, a blended operation with the Department for International Development (United Kingdom) (DFID) and in collaboration with the WHO. As a result, DOTS has expanded to cover more than two-thirds of the country, and there are plans to expand further, resulting in the likely achievement of the Millennium Development Goal target for tuberculosis.

Control of tuberculosis in China is threatened by a large HIV epidemic, undoing many of the gains of the tuberculosis control program. With current high rates of latent tuberculosis, the risk for significant increases in tuberculosis would be enhanced as socially marginalized populations, such as injecting drug users, commercial sex workers, and prisoners, develop AIDS and subsequently tuberculosis as an opportunistic infection. The interaction between HIV/AIDS and tuberculosis is critical in developing strategies for the control of both diseases in China and across the rest of the region.

CHAPTER 2

Current National Responses to HIV/AIDS

At the United Nations General Assembly Special Session on HIV/AIDS in 2001, all EAP countries committed themselves to confronting HIV/AIDS. This commitment was reconfirmed at several regional meetings, including the Seventh Summit of the Association of Southeast Asian Nations (ASEAN) in November 2001. Yet commitments are often difficult to put into practice. To ensure accountability and promote sustainability, commitments must be translated into action. What lessons can be learned to date from efforts to address HIV/AIDS in the EAP Region?

The Thai Experience: Merging Political Commitment, Surveillance, and Civil Society

Thailand illustrates both what has been accomplished in the fight against the epidemic and what still needs to be done.[8] The first country in the region with a generalized HIV/AIDS epidemic, Thailand has shown that a growing epidemic can be controlled through inexpensive, technically simple public health interventions.

The initial response to the epidemic, identified in 1984, was muted. The government believed that the epidemic would remain concentrated in groups practicing high-risk behaviors, particularly injecting drug users and men who have sex with men. This view changed in 1989, when the first national epidemiological surveillance found that 44 percent of sex workers in the northern province of Chiang Mai were infected with HIV, leading first to increasing rates of HIV infection among their male clients and then among the general population.

The Thai Response

Thailand's response was based on political commitment to tackle difficult social issues such as sexual behavior and commercial sex work. The government, including the king and the prime minister, made HIV/AIDS prevention a priority and focused on decreasing high-risk behavior. Four main developments catalyzed political support for confronting HIV/AIDS.

- AIDS policy was put under the Office of the Prime Minister, and the prime minister chaired the multisectoral National AIDS Prevention and Control Committee. This signaled high-level political commitment and opened up dialogue with nongovernmental organizations (NGOs) and other groups.

- A public information campaign was launched with high-level political support from a nationally known political figure with experience in family planning campaigns and strong ties to NGOs.

- HIV prevention among commercial sex workers was introduced. This innovative program provided regular testing of Commercial Sex Workers (CSWs), information and education for both CSWs and their clients, and condom provision. It depended on close cooperation between public health officials and law enforcement.

- A variety of repressive policies were repealed, such as the mandatory reporting of the names and addresses of people with HIV.

The key to the Thai success was effective HIV prevention in CSWs and their clients. The Thai intervention was also grounded in a comprehensive surveillance system. Supported by more than a decade of technical cooperation with the U.S. Centers for Disease Control and Prevention, Thailand had good serological surveillance of the general population, sentinel surveillance of groups whose members practice high-risk behavior, and behavioral surveillance monitoring risky behavior. This surveillance identified some of the key sources of the spread of the disease and monitored the effectiveness of public health interventions. And this public health infrastructure enabled commercial sex workers to receive regular checkups for sexually transmitted infections—infections that can increase the chance of contracting and transmitting HIV.

These prevention programs are associated with a decreased demand for commercial sex, a significant increase in condom use in commercial sex, a decrease in sexually transmitted infections, and ultimately a decrease in new HIV infections. Condom use in brothels rose from about 14 percent to more than 90 percent between 1988 and 1992 (Figure 2). Between 1990 and 1993, the percent of men reporting any premarital and extramarital sex dropped from 28 percent to 15 percent, and the percent visiting sex workers dropped from 22 percent to 10 percent. HIV prevalence among 21-year-old army conscripts, which had risen to 4 percent in 1993, began a steady decline to 1.56 percent by 1999. The decline was even more profound in the North, where it dropped from 12 percent to less than 2 percent. Sexually transmitted infections among men also declined dramatically (Figure 2).

The impact of these interventions on the epidemiology of HIV/AIDS is difficult to quantify. The Asian Epidemic Model predicts that without the interventions there would have been 6.7 million additional infections in Thailand by 2000 (Thai Working Group on HIV/AIDS Projections 2001).

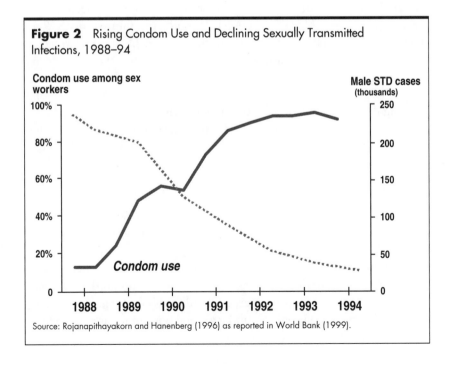

Figure 2 Rising Condom Use and Declining Sexually Transmitted Infections, 1988–94

Condom use among sex workers

Male STD cases (thousands)

Condom use

1988 1989 1990 1991 1992 1993 1994

Source: Rojanapithayakorn and Hanenberg (1996) as reported in World Bank (1999).

The model suggests that public health interventions were responsible for reducing the number of new cases of HIV from 143,000 in 1991 to 29,000 in 2000 (Thai Working Group on HIV/AIDS Projections 2001).[9]

The Thai Experience: Where to Go from Here?

Although Thailand eventually slowed the growth of the epidemic, the high HIV prevalence rates in the past indicate that many people are now developing and dying from AIDS. So Thailand must meet a growing demand for care, support, and treatment. Thailand has an estimated 20,000 patients on antiretroviral therapy, many through unstructured treatment in the private sector, and the number is expected to grow. To prevent the growth in resistance, medical treatment should be standardized, and people living with AIDS should also be treated for opportunistic infections. Treatment is more than medical interventions and should include care and support as well as palliative care for the dying. Finally, because there is a lot we do not know about the interactions between curative and preventive interventions, it is important to maintain vigilant surveillance to understand the potential for recurring growth.

In addition, the HIV prevention agenda is unfinished. Despite the great success, Thailand continues to have high rates of HIV among injecting drug users, a major source of HIV infection that could drive future growth (Reid and Costigan 2002). Short-term substitution therapy has been introduced, but relapse rates are high, and longer-term maintenance therapy is being considered. There are few, if any, needle and syringe exchange programs. Under these circumstances it is likely that HIV will continue to grow among injecting drug users. To prevent this, the government will need to address issues that are extremely stigmatized. HIV prevention programs among men who have sex with men are also limited and would need similar levels of political support.

There is also the chance that the 100 percent condom policy for commercial sex workers could break down. The condom policy is difficult to implement and enforce among "indirect" sex workers.[10] There is also concern because of the significant decrease in HIV prevention funding, particularly after the Asian economic crisis.

As the mature epidemics in Western Europe and North America have shown, high-risk behavior increases as the risk of HIV diminishes, particularly among the young who never experienced the HIV epidemic at its peak. Continued prevention programs in the general population are key to halting the epidemic.

The Cambodian Experience: Using the 100 Percent Condom Policy

Similar to the Thai model, Cambodia has also been successful in decreasing high-risk behavior and slowing the growth of the epidemic (Cambodia Working Group on HIV/AIDS Projection 2002).[11] With Bank support, Cambodia successfully piloted its own version of a 100 percent condom use program in Sihanoukville (under conditions quite different from those in Thailand) and has adopted such a policy nationwide. Condom use among commercial sex workers in areas where the programs have been implemented has risen. Though there has been a recent decline in HIV prevalence, attributing this decline to the 100 percent condom use program is questionable because the pilot was not launched until 1998 and has still not been implemented nationally. Higher mortality may have played a role in the decline in HIV. Regardless, the program shows the importance of a local pilot and demonstrates the feasibility for wider replication that can improve political acceptability.

The decline in HIV was accomplished with limited domestic funding and limited state capacity and supplemented by strong partnerships with international development agencies. Cambodia is a positive example of international development cooperation, linking UNAIDS, WHO, USAID, the Department for International Development (DFID), the Asian Development Bank, and the World Bank in fostering an effective national response to HIV/AIDS.

The Philippines Experience: A Success Story in a Completely Different Context

Another success in the region is the Philippines. In contrast to Thailand's experience, however, its success is found not only in the response to the epidemic, but also in differing commercial sexual practices in the country, emphasizing yet again the diversity in the region. The success story of the Philippines lies in the country's measured response to the epidemic, with national law reform to reduce the likelihood of discrimination, widely available voluntary counseling and testing services, and an adequate number of referral centers for the relatively few people living with HIV/AIDS. There is also a sentinel and behavioral surveillance system. However, the main factors constraining the epidemic in the Philippines appear to have less to do with prevention programs and more to do with contextual factors—for example, commercial sex workers have few sexual partners, there are high rates of circumcision, and there are low levels of injecting drug use and ulcerative sexually transmitted infections.

Although the epidemic is classified as low level, the Philippines must continue to invest in and improve public health surveillance. Currently, the sample sizes for surveillance are smaller than optimal for detecting changes in the general population. There are high levels of certain sexually transmitted infections in the population, and sexual behaviors appear to be changing (Philippines Department of Health 2002).

The Indonesian Experience: The Importance of Political Commitment in Low-Level Epidemics

In 1996 the government of Indonesia, recognizing the importance of early intervention in preventing an epidemic, developed and funded an HIV/AIDS and sexually transmitted infections program, which included some funding from several donors, including the World Bank. HIV was reported in men who have sex with men and transvestites, and there was high-risk behavior among commercial sex workers. The program focused on building surveillance capacity and expanding interventions to commercial sex workers and the general population. But the World Bank portion was closed in 1999 after the Asian economic crisis, disbursing only $4.52 million of $24.8 million allocated.

There are many lessons from the HIV/AIDS project in Indonesia. The economic crisis played an important role, as the health sector was preoccupied with the immediate crisis. Pharmaceutical availability was severely affected and prices rose dramatically, and large increases in poverty threatened to overwhelm an already overburdened public health system (see Box 2 for a discussion of health sector capacity).

Another contributing factor was limited government capacity. Responsibility for HIV/AIDS was spread throughout the Ministry of Health, with limited coordination across units. There was also inadequate capacity in the NGO sector. NGOs were generally too small and without the necessary experience to carry out complex interventions. Capacity for surveillance activities, particularly behavioral surveillance, was also limited, though the project did develop laboratory infrastructure for surveillance. As HIV prevalence remained low and the predicted epidemic did not materialize, sustaining the political commitment to develop innovative multisectoral interventions for vulnerable groups became more difficult.

Box 2 Interactions Between HIV/AIDS and the Capacity of Health Systems: SARS as a Case Study

In several countries in the region, HIV/AIDS is straining health systems. Health systems in many of these countries already lack capacity and are overburdened—a major concern for countries with generalized epidemics, because demand for health services increases as people develop AIDS. It should also be a concern for countries with concentrated epidemics, because they need to look toward building infrastructure and capacity to care for the sick and dying.

A different, recent epidemic illustrates this point. The outbreak of severe acute respiratory syndrome (SARS) illustrated the critical importance of public health systems and surveillance, including accurate reporting on new cases and deaths. Health systems were overwhelmed by an influx of sick and dying people, quickly realizing that they lacked the capacity to deal with the disease. The short time between contact with the disease and death heightened fears and created panic, highlighting the need to create systems that can both allay fears and accurately report on the number of cases. The lag time between contact and the development of symptoms for AIDS is much longer, but the disease places similar strains on health systems, calling for actions to increase capacity.

Over the years, the epidemiology of HIV/AIDS in Indonesia has changed. HIV/AIDS is now concentrated among injecting drug users and, in some places, more than 60 percent of injecting drug users are HIV-positive. HIV prevalence is also growing among commercial sex workers. HIV prevention among injecting drug users is very limited, and there is no 100 percent condom policy.

More recently, government commitment appears to be increasing, with a new HIV/AIDS strategy embracing HIV prevention in groups whose members practice high-risk behavior. Indonesia has also introduced a good epidemiological surveillance system. Mounting an effective response will remain a challenge for Indonesia in the coming years.

The Papua New Guinea Experience: A Different Epidemic

Papua New Guinea (PNG) is at risk for developing a large, heterosexual HIV/AIDS epidemic that might even follow the trajectory of the disease in Sub-Saharan Africa. Together the breakdown of traditional methods of social control in PNG, the cash economy, urbanization, and greater mobility have resulted in very significant changes in sexual behavior. These factors, combined with a health system that lacks capacity to deal with even basic preventive care, place the country at significant risk.

HIV was first reported in PNG in 1987. From the mid-1990s onwards the epidemic started to grow quickly. Despite numerous alerts raised in the early 1990s to the emerging epidemic, few persons in positions of leadership acknowledged HIV/AIDS as an issue of concern. With encouragement and funds from the Global Program on AIDS (GPA), the National AIDS Program was formed and enlisted membership from a wide variety of stakeholders into a National AIDS Committee. These and other efforts, however, were difficult to sustain. The National AIDS Committee functioned only sporadically from 1988 to 1994, and efforts in the early 1990s to establish a sentinel surveillance system faltered and by 1995 all that remained was limited passive surveillance in some locations. In 1997 a new government response emerged, and a Medium-Term Plan (MTP) was constructed to cover 1998–2002. The multisectoral approach and objectives of the MTP, however, were never operationalized, costed, prioritized, or implemented. All targeted interventions were disbanded and became imbedded in a planned, but unimplemented, national peer education program. A recent review of the implementation of the MTP reveals only limited success to date.

Although the total resources available for the response to HIV/AIDS in Papua New Guinea are high (well in excess of $8 million; more than $1.60 per person per capita in 2003–04), commitment of the PNG government, the nature of the response, and the quality of the interventions are in question. There is a heavy bias toward interventions in urban areas, although more than half, and as much as three-quarters, of the infected people are in rural areas. Implementation is poor and hampered by a severe lack of human resources. Targeted prevention efforts (for people practicing high-risk behaviors), quality sentinel surveillance, and monitoring and evaluation of interventions are urgently needed to ameliorate the possible negative impacts of this epidemic.

Other Countries Facing Similar Challenges

It would be a difficult task to define the depth and breadth of lessons learned in all countries throughout the region. The examples given, however, show the broad range of experiences, highlighting some important lessons. Prevention, surveillance, and political commitment can have an impact. A strong response is needed in low-level epidemics. And care must be taken as society and values evolve. The concentrated epidemics of China, Vietnam, and Malaysia also exhibit a mixed fare of projects, responses, and inputs. Unfortunately, however, there is strong potential for HIV/AIDS growth in all of these countries.

China's emerging epidemic is considered to be the next big challenge on the horizon. HIV and AIDS cases are increasing, and there is spread from high-risk populations to the general population (China MOH/UNAIDS 2003). One of the lessons from China is the importance of the blood supply. China has made progress in moving toward a system of voluntary blood donations and creating the infrastructure necessary to ensure the safety of the blood supply. In addition, the Chinese central government recently reaffirmed its commitment to achieving the United Nations General Assembly Special Session on HIV/AIDS (UNGASS) goals. It plans to improve laws and regulations, to launch public awareness campaigns, to protect the rights of people living with HIV/AIDS, to increase international cooperation on HIV/AIDS, and to provide antiretrovirals.

Many other countries have created similar national AIDS strategies. For example, Vietnam recently completed its national strategy. But action is what is now needed. The way these and other strategies and lessons are adopted and adapted within the East Asia Region will determine the future of the epidemic and the social and economic landscape of Asian society.

CHAPTER 3

Key Challenges

To combat the epidemic, five key challenges must be addressed:

- Political commitment and multisectoral support
- Public health surveillance and monitoring and evaluation
- Prevention
- Care, support, and treatment
- Health services delivery.

Political Commitment and Multisectoral Support

Given the sensitive nature of the disease, political commitment is key to effective HIV/AIDS programs, as Thailand and Cambodia have shown. HIV prevention programs are difficult to implement because they often involve sexual and drug-using behaviors governed by complex social taboos. An important aspect to facilitating dialogue and making progress around these issues is building political understanding by promoting public awareness of HIV/AIDS prevention programs.

Gaining political commitment for prevention in low-level epidemics, as in Indonesia in the 1990s, can be extremely difficult. One lesson is the importance of having the ministry of health actively engaged and well organized. In Indonesia, where responsibility for HIV/AIDS was spread across the ministry of health, coordination was weak. In Thailand, where the HIV/AIDS program was run out of the high-profile office of the prime minister, the high level and visibility of political commitment helped to open dialogue with NGOs and other sectors.

Effective prevention also requires a social response beyond the health sector. A multisectoral response requires political commitment to implement HIV prevention in groups with high-risk behaviors, such as commercial sex workers, injecting drug users, and men who have sex with men. It often requires changes in legislation to allow active prevention and outreach programs to reach these hidden populations, activities rarely provided by traditional public health services. And it also requires active collaboration with law enforcement agencies, as well as nongovernmental organizations.

As the epidemic spreads and generalizes, care, support, and treatment become important elements of HIV/AIDS programming. When many people are living with AIDS, support services are required from a variety of sectors in addition to health, based on the needs of the country and the stage of the epidemic.

It is also important to better understand the role of NGOs, civil society, cultural figures, champions, and key leaders. More analysis of their roles is needed to gain a better understanding of how to improve outcomes.

In addition, there is a need to guard the human rights of individuals at risk of acquiring the virus and those living with the virus. Many people do not have appropriate access to services, prevention messages, care, support, or treatment. Individuals living with the virus face rejection from their family, friends, and society. To combat stigma, many governments have responded by passing laws against discrimination and expanding access to treatment. Political commitment to face this issue will be a major key to successful initiatives.

The World Bank has several comparative advantages in working in these arenas in the EAP Region. First, it works broadly across sectors and can bring together all parts of government for policy dialogue, including the ministries of finance, health, planning, and education. It can also play an important role in donor coordination. Although political commitment and multisectorality are key to an effective response, the important sectors and appropriate government involvement vary by the needs of the country, the stage of the epidemic, and the nature of the groups that practice high-risk behaviors.

Public Health Surveillance and Monitoring and Evaluation

Although much is known about HIV/AIDS in the East Asia and Pacific Region, more is unknown. To date, there are few good estimates of the size of populations practicing high-risk behaviors, such as commercial sex workers and injecting drug users—essential for estimating the potential growth of the epidemic. It is also necessary to know how these sex workers and drug-using populations overlap. Multiple approaches may be needed to understand the potential for growth of HIV/AIDS in a society and the effectiveness of interventions. These include routine information collection systems, including surveys and qualitative research. More funding is needed for public health surveillance and social science research on sexual and drug-using behaviors, along with increased capacity for conducting research in local universities and government agencies. Also important is linking routine information datasets from health, criminal justice, and social services.

The importance of various components of public health surveillance varies with the stage of the epidemic. In low-level epidemics, it is very important to understand the size of high-risk populations and the prevalence of high-risk behavior to determine the potential for growth. This requires national behavioral studies and good sociocultural studies with rapid situational assessments that can be complemented by good sentinel and behavioral surveillance systems.

Surveillance becomes even more important in concentrated epidemics, where there are relatively high rates of HIV/AIDS among populations with high-risk behaviors. In these situations, it is important to standardize the methodology for sentinel surveillance and to link it to behavioral surveillance. China, Indonesia, and Vietnam have sentinel surveillance systems. Though sociocultural studies on risk behavior are limited, there are some good examples. Indonesia recently carried out a multimethod study on the size of at-risk populations, and this study could be replicated throughout the region.[12]

Sentinel surveillance in groups whose members practice high-risk behaviors is also important in generalized epidemics, but surveillance must also be extended to the general population, through regular monitoring of HIV in antenatal clinics, sexually transmitted infection clinics, and the blood supply. It is also useful to have other proxies for the general population. When an epidemic is generalized, sexually transmitted infections and tuberculosis become even more important, and there should be good general surveillance of both in the general population. In late generalized epidemics, as increasing numbers of people develop AIDS, the need arises for a good reporting system, the ability to monitor the blood count of AIDS patients, and the capacity to monitor drug resistance.

Surveillance helps to understand the nature of the problem and to identify solutions. This requires extending surveillance beyond diseases to monitoring and evaluating whether interventions have achieved their desired goals, such as reducing risk behavior and decreasing the incidence of HIV/AIDS, and applying the findings to prevention programs. Achieving a significant decrease in high-risk behavior requires large-scale social programs that reach a substantial proportion of the targeted population. Only if these programs are widespread will they have an impact on the epidemiology of HIV/AIDS. Monitoring must ensure that care, support, and treatment improve life expectancy, reach the poor, and minimize drug resistance. It also requires improving routine health information systems to measure coverage of prevention and treatment programs, health outcomes, and financial costs.

Prevention

On the global level, fewer than one in five individuals at risk of HIV infection has access to basic prevention services. In Asia, with combinations of drug use, unprotected sex, and rising rates of sexually transmitted infections, UNAIDS estimates that only 10 percent or fewer of injecting drug users and other vulnerable populations are benefiting from prevention interventions (Global HIV Prevention Working Group 2003). Still, there have been some major successes in this arena within the region. Thailand and Cambodia have demonstrated the cost-effectiveness of HIV prevention among commercial sex workers and their clients through the 100 percent condom policy. But this is not a panacea. UNAIDS notes that the HIV/AIDS epidemic can be slowed if prevention programs such as these are scaled up and used in combination with other prevention efforts to target groups affected by HIV/AIDS and the diverse routes of transmission (Global HIV Prevention Working Group 2003).

Another important public health approach, especially in the EAP Region, is to reduce risky behavior among injecting drug users and thus HIV transmission. This has been shown to be possible in many countries with concentrated HIV/AIDS epidemics among injecting drug users, such as Australia, Canada, Germany, Netherlands, Switzerland, and United Kingdom. They applied an inclusive policy, called harm reduction, that recognizes drug use as an addiction and uses active social outreach to bring injecting drug users into contact with HIV/AIDS preventive services and drug treatment. Instead of harm reduction policies, some governments have pursued policies aimed at eliminating drug use, but from a public health standpoint, eradicating

HIV/AIDS from the drug-using population is probably easier than eliminating drug use.

There is broad scope for improving HIV prevention in injecting drug users. This is clearly an important issue on the HIV prevention agenda for the East Asia and Pacific Region. Drug treatment services are poorly developed and substitution therapy is almost nonexistent.[13] But there has been some change. Hong Kong, China, has an internationally recognized drug treatment system. In Indonesia a pilot project for harm reduction in Bali has been adopted by the Ministry of Health as national policy, though it has yet to be implemented.

As noted above, one successful element of the Thai effort to prevent the spread of HIV was to improve the management of sexually transmitted infections in groups whose behaviors place them at risk. There is currently an epidemic of sexually transmitted infections in the region. This is important in and of itself, but also suggests there is strong potential for growth of HIV/AIDS in the region.[14] The ability of sexually transmitted infections to fuel the HIV epidemic could be alarming, especially in countries like China and Indonesia. Treatment of sexually transmitted infections is a critical component of prevention.

Another important group that needs to be addressed is youth. In 1999 half of the world's 15,000 new daily infections occurred among 15- to 24-year-olds (World Bank 2002). Because youth—and other subgroups—can engage in several risky behaviors, they may be an important entry point for prevention. A related concern is young women. Women, and young women in particular, often have less bargaining power in sexual relationships, and are therefore more vulnerable to infection. This gender dimension should be addressed in prevention efforts. Other groups, such as migrant laborers, prisoners, and men having sex with men, also need to be targeted as part of prevention strategies and programs.

In most of the preceding situations where prevention is necessary, including those involving youth, education is key. Information, education, and communication campaigns for the general public and high-risk groups are important components of an effective HIV/AIDS prevention strategy. There is also a need for a broader educational approach to prevention that includes the education sector.

Another significant element of prevention is voluntary counseling and testing, which can be important for prevention for both HIV-positive and HIV-negative individuals. Knowledge of their status can assist individuals in making decisions about protecting themselves and their partners. Limited access to voluntary counseling and testing, as well as stigma and discrimination, however, can limit the effectiveness of this intervention. In order to provide these services, discrimination must be addressed. Similarly, the services should be provided in the context of comprehensive health and social systems and targeted to marginalized and hard-to-reach groups.

Care, Support, and Treatment

Care, support, and treatment activities aim to improve the quality of life of individuals and communities affected by HIV/AIDS, while boosting prevention efforts to prevent its further spread. A comprehensive plan of care and support includes diagnosis, treatment, referral and follow-up, nursing care, counseling, and support to meet psychological, spiritual, economic, social, and legal needs. Treatment with pharmaceutical drugs, including antiretroviral therapy, is also important (UNAIDS/WHO/International HIV/AIDS Alliance 2003).

Demand for antiretroviral therapy is growing. To maximize the effectiveness of drug treatment, it should be complemented by care and support and implemented using standardized evidence-based clinical protocols. Implementing these protocols requires strengthening health systems, including improving clinical training, laboratory infrastructure, logistical systems to deliver medicines, and sustainable systems for funding clinical services that are delivering antiretrovirals.

The uptake of antiretroviral therapy varies considerably across the region. Thailand, with its more mature epidemic, has the greatest number of patients on combination therapy. It recently declared its intention to provide universal access to antiretroviral therapy,[15] and has its own generic drug manufacturing system.[16] Cambodia, by contrast, had only about 100 patients in official therapy programs (Calmette hospital) in 2002, while NGOs supported more than 750 patients in pilot studies in Phnom Penh and Siem Reap. In coming years, more patients are expected to receive treatment through the French program Ensemble pur une Solidarité Thérapeutique Hospitalière en Réseau and the expansion of NGO activities (Médecins Sans Frontières, Center of Hope, and Médecins du Monde). Most of them will still be in Phnom Penh and Siem Reap, but it is expected that expansion into Kompong Cham and Takeo Provinces might be possible. In most other countries, there are a limited number of patients on antiretroviral therapy (Gold and Smith 2003).

Antiretroviral therapy is also very important in preventing mother-to-child transmission. Successful prevention programs for mother-to-child transmission require a mixture of prevention, care, support, and treatment, including voluntary counseling and testing, replacement feeding, and antiretroviral therapy (FHI/USAID 2001b).

Moreover, managing HIV infection requires a range of other services including clinical management of HIV/AIDS-related illnesses, prevention and control of opportunistic infections (for example, tuberculosis), palliative care, home care, and psychosocial support. Tuberculosis, as the most common opportunistic infection of HIV/AIDS, is an important disease to target. Though fueled by the HIV/AIDS epidemic, tuberculosis does not confine itself to HIV-positive individuals. When targeting tuberculosis, coordination of tuberculosis and HIV/AIDS services is important.

Support is also necessary for families and dependents of people living with HIV/AIDS. As adults succumb to the disease, more children become orphans. Comprehensive systems of care need to be developed for these orphans, ensuring that they have people to take care of their emotional and financial needs, so that they can continue their educations and receive medical treatment. Programs and policies must be specific to each country's safety nets and varying cultural and social mores.

Voluntary counseling and testing is another component of care and support. Because HIV infection can be asymptomatic for many years, people with HIV who might benefit from early drug treatment are often unaware that they are infected. Voluntary counseling and testing helps arrange for early clinical management of HIV infection before it progresses to AIDS (World Bank 2000). Such programs should first be targeted to groups whose behaviors place them at highest risk, unless there is a generalized epidemic.

Strengthening Health Services Delivery

Most prevention, care, support, and treatment services can be provided by a combination of public health services and social care systems such as hospitals, clinics, and dispensaries, including the private sector and nongovernmental organizations. While some needs can be met outside the health system, much of the disease burden of HIV/AIDS is borne by health systems—hospital and clinical services, laboratory diagnostic support, delivery of pharmaceuticals, maternal-child health services, voluntary counseling and testing services, and palliative and home-based care.

Most people at risk of HIV infection or already infected live in resource-constrained settings. Many health facilities in these settings lack the resources to provide quality health care to the general population, much less meet the complex demands of HIV/AIDS-related morbidity and mortality. Additionally, given that there are going to be increased resources coming into countries through the Global Fund to Fight AIDS, Tuberculosis, and Malaria (GFATM) and other donors, this will increase the strain on already burdened health and social service systems, as well as the broader government. Capacity needs to be strengthened and built within health—and broader—systems if countries are going to scale-up prevention, care, support, and treatment.

Private sector involvement is critical for engaging with HIV/AIDS in the EAP Region. In general, the private sector plays a key role in the delivery of clinical care in the region (Gold and Smith 2003). Much of sexually transmitted infection care is also privately provided, causing significant problems of inappropriate and inadequate care. Scaling-up access to care, support, and treatment requires an innovative approach by and with the private sector. Additionally, as with prevention, public health services rarely reach socially marginalized groups. It is important to develop and strengthen NGOs and other sectors to reach marginal populations.

At the heart of any health system are resources: where they come from, how and on what they are spent, and how effectively they are used. Accounting for resources in this way is not well developed for health systems in general, but is especially poor for HIV/AIDS. It is, however, similar to the more standardized national health accounts used by the Organisation for Economic Co-operation and Development (OECD), the World Health Organization (WHO), and the World Bank. These accounts need to be developed to track overall domestic public spending in health on public goods such as surveillance and prevention among groups with high-risk behaviors. The national health accounts framework also emphasizes understanding private household spending, which is particularly important for HIV/AIDS, given the high levels of private treatment.

CHAPTER 4

The World Bank Strategy for HIV/AIDS in the East Asia and Pacific Region

Lessons from the World Bank over the Last Decade

The World Bank is one of the leading financiers of HIV/AIDS prevention and control activities in the world. It has committed $1.77 billion (and disbursed nearly $800 million) on more than 70 current and future projects around the world. Between 1992 and 2002 the World Bank financed 11 health projects with HIV/AIDS-related components in seven EAP countries. Cumulative lending in the region for HIV/AIDS stands at over $100 million, making the World Bank the largest single financier of HIV/AIDS projects in the region. Nonetheless, World Bank support for the region's health sector makes up only 5.7 percent of the $2.1 billion portfolio of World Bank lending in the EAP Region (Box 3).

Of the 11 projects in the region on HIV/AIDS that the Bank has financed to date, only two have been exclusively for HIV/AIDS: Indonesia HIV/AIDS and STD Prevention and Management Project ($25 million), closed in 1999, and the Vietnam Blood Supply Management Project ($38.2 million). The other projects either included HIV/AIDS as part of an infectious disease project, a maternal health project, or a broader health systems project. The most significant financial support has been in China, with a small HIV/AIDS component in Health V (Infectious and Endemic Disease Control) and VII

37

Box 3 How Much Will It Cost to Prevent the Spread of HIV/AIDS in the EAP Region?

The short answer? We don't know. UNAIDS and the London School of Hygiene and Tropical Medicine estimated that at least $9.2 billion annually is required to mount an appropriate response, including substantial funding for antiretroviral therapy. This estimate is for a basic program of prevention, care, support, and treatment in all developing countries and does not include the cost of improving the health infrastructure. For the EAP Region, they estimated 10 percent of the total, with the majority of funding allocated for prevention ($810 million) and $80 million for care and support (Schwarlander and others 1999). Such a general estimate is not very meaningful at the country level, since it should be based on effective strategies for each country supported by detailed costing. However, even with limited knowledge of the resources needed, it is likely there will be resource gaps in some countries in the region.

So how much is currently being spent? Although the data on domestic spending are sparse, it is clear that public funding for HIV/AIDS is not very significant, with a few exceptions like Thailand. Looking at overall public spending on health shows little room for spending on HIV/AIDS. In most countries, it is less than 1 percent of public spending, meaning that the region is far from the estimate of need. Of course, most of the money spent on HIV/AIDS may not come from public expenditures, but through private household spending. The spread of AIDS is likely to increase private expenditures significantly as households pay for antiretroviral therapy and care, and as they try to absorb the loss of income due to inability to work.

With low levels of government spending on HIV/AIDS, international development assistance has become a large player in this arena.

(Health Promotion) Projects, culminating in $25.6 million for HIV/AIDS prevention and control in Health IX.

Although the projects differ based on country needs, they share some common elements, particularly the strengthening of national and provincial surveillance systems. All projects include health promotion to the general population and groups whose members practice high-risk behaviors, though earlier projects gave more emphasis to health services capacity. More recent projects tend to be more comprehensive, though issues of care and support for HIV/AIDS are addressed only in China Health IX. All projects attempt to build multisectoral involvement, including NGOs, but effectiveness appears to be mixed.

Overall, the projects tended to be stronger on technical design than on implementation. The most effective components were related to hardware—improving the laboratory network for HIV/AIDS and sexually transmitted infections in Indonesia or blood safety in China. (Additional information on blood safety in countries in the region is available in Annex 7). Limited national and provincial government capacity has impacted implementation effectiveness. Channeling funds and contracting with NGOs were concerns for some of these projects in earlier project designs. Inadequate monitoring and evaluation systems and capacity also affected programming.

Analytic and advisory work within the region is becoming a more important component of the World Bank response to HIV/AIDS. A seminal document on HIV/AIDS, *Thailand Social Monitor: Thailand's Response to AIDS: Building on Success, Confronting the Future* (World Bank 2000) fully explains the epidemic in Thailand and identifies areas of strategic priority. There are a number of new pieces of analytic work underway in several countries, including Indonesia, Thailand, and China, and demand appears to be increasing.

Lessons Learned

Lessons from the Bank's activities include the following:

- More analytic and advisory work is needed to support HIV/AIDS programs in the region and to provide the basis for financing/lending activities.

- The Bank needs to pay closer attention to monitoring and evaluation across the health sector, especially in view of the increased emphasis on results.

- Because insufficient capacity may cause even well designed projects to fail, the implementation capacity of national HIV/AIDS programs and NGOs needs to be enhanced. Innovation in project design to support NGOs and local governments, and to channel funds for multisectoral work, would help improve implementation.

- The Bank has the capacity to work across sectors and incorporate HIV/AIDS components into a range of development projects (infrastructure, education projects).

- The Bank is well placed to work across the health sector and to strengthen health services delivery.

- With the increased emphasis on partnerships, different models to support HIV/AIDS work can be developed.

World Bank in Relation to Other Donors

Because the groups involved in the fight against HIV/AIDS have been changing rapidly, it is important to review the sources of support to identify gaps and decrease duplication. Though the World Bank is one of the region's largest single financiers of HIV/AIDS programs, it will soon be displaced by the GFATM, which has committed over $400 million for the next 5 years. Set up in January 2002 to provide complementary financing to existing programs addressing HIV/AIDS, tuberculosis, and malaria, the GFATM seeks to attract, manage, and disburse additional resources to scale-up interventions and treatment through a new public-private partnership. To date the GFATM has had three rounds of proposals with total commitments of over $2.0 billion (Annex 8).

The role of the GFATM in providing resources for HIV/AIDS is likely to have implications for the World Bank. The GFATM serves primarily as a financing mechanism. The implication of this for countries is that implementation and technical assistance have to be provided by someone else, for example, bilaterals, the Bank, and other donors. In addition, there are likely to be issues surrounding how the funds are used and whether countries have the capacity to implement large-scale programs of prevention and treatment and to monitor and evaluate the results.

Another key player is the UNAIDS Secretariat, whose main purpose is to act as a catalyst and coordinator of action on HIV/AIDS, rather than as a direct funding or implementing agency. UNAIDS is playing a greater role in coordination and advocacy, including tracking international development assistance on HIV/AIDS, setting global standards for monitoring and evaluation, and tracking the HIV/AIDS epidemic. At the country level, UNAIDS is the convener of the U.N. family through the UNAIDS theme group that aims to help countries mount an effective multisectoral response to HIV/AIDS.

The World Health Organization is playing an increasingly larger role in HIV/AIDS. They are the main source of technical guidance in areas such as diagnosis and treatment of sexually transmitted infections, care, treatment, and support of AIDS, prevention, and the interaction between HIV/AIDS and tuberculosis. Recently the WHO launched a new strategy aimed at increasing access to treatment (3 by 5 Initiative).

Bilateral agencies [for example, USAID, the Australian government's overseas aid program (AusAID), DFID, and Japan International Cooperation Agency (JICA)] are in the forefront of interventions among populations whose members practice high-risk behaviors. AusAID is supporting harm reduction in China, Indonesia, Myanmar, and Vietnam, and DFID in China. These programs are generally limited in scope, but serve as models that could be replicated by governments. USAID plays a large role in developing capacity for epidemiological surveillance, particularly behavioral surveillance. The U.S. Centers for Disease Control and Prevention (CDC) have partnered with the Thai CDC for more than a decade and have been instrumental in building capacity in epidemiological surveillance in the Untied States, China, and Vietnam.

There are several regional initiatives working in HIV/AIDS as well, including the Asian Development Bank's program for the Mekong Delta. Other agencies are also working regionally: USAID is reopening a regional office in Thailand, and UNAIDS, the WHO, UNICEF, and the United Nations Office on Drugs and Crime (UNODC) are major regional players. The Association of Southeast Asian Nations (ASEAN) is working on a five-year plan to combat HIV/AIDS in mobile populations, including seafarers, truck drivers, and migrant workers.

The World Bank also has a separate and specific role in the region. Specifically, as a co-convenor of multiple sectors, the World Bank has the opportunity to bring together a number of players to discuss—and take action on—HIV/AIDS, in collaboration with governments and other partners, including UNAIDS. In addition, the long-term presence of the World Bank in countries and its multisectoral lending program can help address long-term systemic issues. Even in an era of increased grant funding through the GFATM and other bilaterals, the World Bank may play an important role in resource mobilization for HIV/AIDS.

Strategic Directions

The World Bank strategy will respond to these challenges by developing country-specific strategies based on the needs of the country and the stage of the epidemic in the country. These HIV/AIDS country strategy notes will be the basis for World Bank engagement. They will also be designed in concert with national strategic HIV/AIDS plans created by governments and the World Bank Country Assistance Strategies. These HIV/AIDS strategy notes will provide specific work plans that incorporate some mix of the following tools: analytic and advisory work, lending, and regional activities. And they will be designed to be flexible and innovative, focusing on the following five key challenges.

Political Commitment and Multisectoral Support

The experience from Thailand, Cambodia, and other countries that have been successful in tackling HIV/AIDS shows the need for strong leadership and a coordinated multisectoral response. More analytic work is needed to understand how the World Bank can increase political commitment across a broad spectrum of sectors and, with it, public awareness of HIV/AIDS. Analytic work will help identify key stakeholders, their institutional setting, and the barriers to political commitment. It will also help identify the key sectors and help the Bank better integrate multisectoral approaches into work at the country level.

Communications are also necessary for building political understanding and commitment across a broad sectoral spectrum (health, education, transport) and for increasing public support for HIV/AIDS prevention programs. For example, the Eastern Europe and Central Asia Region is planning to use public opinion surveys to understand not only *what* people think, but *why*, and to identify their underlying motivations and biases about HIV/AIDS. Such understanding is critical to ensuring that communication aimed at achieving political commitment, raising awareness, and changing attitudes and behaviors is focused and resonates with critical audiences. A similar method could be used in East Asia, providing a resource for country and sectoral teams working on HIV/AIDS issues and for client governments to gain a better understanding of stakeholder perceptions and the environment in which they operate.

Public Health Surveillance and Monitoring and Evaluation

Public health surveillance. All countries in the EAP Region need to improve their public health surveillance systems, a public good that tends to be underfunded. Improved HIV/AIDS surveillance includes HIV sentinel surveillance, behavioral surveillance, and sociocultural studies to determine the size and overlap of high-risk populations. The work can build on good models for surveillance that already exist in the region. In addition, support and resources to implement these systems and build capacity are needed.

Within surveillance, better HIV/AIDS projections are needed. To help governments design and prioritize programs, it is important to understand the future course of the epidemic under various hypotheses. Understanding the socioeconomic consequences of HIV/AIDS requires better data for epidemiological projections. Projections and operations research are also needed to assist governments in planning for the burden of HIV-related diseases, including tuberculosis. For example, the Cambodia tuberculosis program has worked with the National Center for HIV/AIDS, Dermatology, and STDs to project cases of HIV-related tuberculosis and to develop decentralized services to handle the increases in tuberculosis. This requires assessing the increased demand for health spending and then developing actual models of service delivery.

Socioeconomic impact models are also needed to understand the effect of HIV/AIDS on the health care system, household, and macroeconomy. Other models would also help in understanding the links between human development and poverty by analyzing the effects of HIV/AIDS on the household. Such models would combine epidemiological projection models and household survey data on income and consumption.

Monitoring and evaluation. In the EAP Region, monitoring and evaluation are likely to play a central role in the World Bank strategy, possibly involving national health accounts for HIV/AIDS and monitoring of the coverage of interventions. To ensure sustainable domestic financing for HIV/AIDS for scaling-up interventions, governments first need to better understand the current level of spending. Analytic and advisory work could help governments track public expenditures for HIV/AIDS using a national health accounts framework. This is currently being done in Indonesia and Cambodia and could be expanded across the region. The analysis should include private spending on HIV/AIDS prevention and treatment. This type of accounting is not well developed for HIV/AIDS, but is similar to that used in standard national health accounts. But tracking public spending on almost any social program in the EAP Region is difficult and related to public sector management and reforms.

Monitoring and evaluation require more than expenditure tracking—they also require systems to determine whether interventions are reaching the target population at adequate coverage, especially for the poor. Many of these systems are weak and need to be improved. Where routine information systems are unreliable, techniques such as household surveys and sentinel sites will be needed. The World Bank can work with governments to develop and implement monitoring and evaluation plans to track an effective response.

Prevention

The key to effective prevention programs is reaching high enough coverage levels among high-risk populations to have an epidemiological impact. Though many countries have successful pilot projects, they have very limited coverage. Many of these interventions are politically difficult, such as prevention among injecting drug users and commercial sex workers, but are necessary and require strong political commitment. A first step would be to pull together all the epidemiological and financial information into a coherent system. A second step would be to look at the resources needed for scaling-up related to human resources and financing.

In some countries, the World Bank might also play a role in improving information on high-risk behavior and building capacity for behavioral research. Understanding sex workers and injecting drug users and their overlap is important for estimating growth of the epidemic and for preparing effective interventions. But in most countries the information on sex workers and injecting drug users that is needed to design effective prevention programs is limited. In addition, political support and ensuring that there are adequate resources for prevention programs are key for addressing the HIV/AIDS epidemic. Again, depending on the country strategy and demand, the World Bank can play an important role.

Care, Support, and Treatment

Treatment of AIDS with antiretroviral therapy is occurring in almost all countries in the EAP Region and is likely to increase, particularly as donor support for treatment programs increases. Analytic work is needed to understand how to increase treatment in the context of relatively weak systems of service delivery. Options might include using existing platforms of care, such as tuberculosis programs, to expand treatment with antiretroviral therapy. It is essential to engage with the private sector, because this is often where treatment is already occurring. Also treatment must be embedded within a larger system of care and support, including treatment of opportunistic infections, links between treatment and prevention, and care for the dying.

Health Services Delivery

Many health systems in the region are going through a transition. There is limited capacity in the public and private sectors and an important role for the nongovernmental sector, including the private sector, in service delivery. A better understanding of health system issues, opportunities, and constraints is essential for many HIV/AIDS interventions. While the exact type of work needed can be determined only at the individual country level, some examples could include funding public health interventions and surveillance under decentralization; integrating the private sector and NGOs for HIV/AIDS prevention and treatment; integrating health and social services, particularly for groups whose members practice high-risk behaviors; improving the laboratory infrastructure for testing and treatment of HIV/AIDS; enhancing the safety of the blood supply; and building capacity in general, especially for care, support, and treatment. There will also need to be a focus on how to increase absorptive capacity within health systems as well as within the broader government.

Additionally, the World Bank has been playing an important role in health systems development in several countries in the region. In the same way, the World Bank can assist governments in preparing health systems to deal with HIV/AIDS. Also, as many of these interventions require multisectoral activities and interventions, assisting with health systems issues in decentralized settings is another important area in which, together with the other partners, the World Bank may be able to provide support.

As stated, these key challenges will be addressed through specific work plans that incorporate some mix of the tools described in the following sections.

Analytic and Advisory Work

Analytic and advisory work assists the World Bank in carrying on policy dialogue with governments and civil society on an effective response to HIV/AIDS. The focus will vary based on the needs of the country and region, the role of government and other partners, and the stage of the epidemic. Analytic and advisory work will support all of the key challenges as part of an effective HIV/AIDS strategy in the region.

As countries face various policy options, the World Bank has traditionally played an important role in this arena that can be expanded to include HIV/AIDS. Of course, the range of advisory and analytic work is wide and depends on country needs.

Lending and Funding for HIV/AIDS in the EAP Region

The International Development Association (IDA) can provide credits and/or grants for HIV/AIDS programs in IDA-eligible countries, while in middle-income International Bank for Reconstruction and Development (IBRD) countries, where grant funding is limited, there is an important role for partnerships with other development organizations. The exact demand for World Bank funding is hard to predict since it is a function of many variables, including the availability of domestic funding and grants. But there are clear areas in which governments have a role and in which there is a general pattern of underinvestment—areas that may represent a priority for World Bank support. For instance, many countries in the region could benefit from improvements in public health surveillance and monitoring and evaluation. These could require a combination of investments in routine information systems and research, hardware, software, and technical assistance. The World Bank stands ready to support both analytic and lending programs in countries in the region, depending on specific country needs and demands.

Equally important is determining how the World Bank can be more effective in providing financial support for HIV/AIDS programs whether through lending or grants. Some of this may require a different way of doing business. Different options are needed for designing multisectoral projects, for channeling funds and building capacity of NGOs, for including the private sector, and for building monitoring and evaluation systems. With the introduction in recent years of more flexible designs and more options for addressing client needs and demands, there is room for more effective programs—programs that take into account the key lessons from the first cohort of projects.

Regional Activities

Where there is value added from cross-country experience or from country-specific interventions and analysis, a regional role for the World Bank might be appropriate, especially in support for public health surveillance and monitoring and evaluation.

Regional Tools

A number of areas were identified in which sharing experiences and tools could be helpful, such as experiences with implementation of national accounts for HIV/AIDS. Improvements in such areas could be facilitated by the development of new tools that are regional in scope but adapted to each country's needs. Examples include improved projection models for HIV/AIDS, socioeconomic models of the impact of HIV/AIDS, optimization models of public spending, and other similar tools.

Regional Dissemination of Best Practice

The World Bank will work with partners, especially UNAIDS and the World Bank Institute, to disseminate best practice in HIV/AIDS prevention and control throughout the region. Thailand implemented an effective prevention program among commercial sex workers and a strong surveillance system. This is an example of an experience that can be shared more broadly in the region.

A related and important point is that the World Bank, with its ability to work across sectors, can help build support and share knowledge through its convening role. The Bank will work in close partnerships on a regional level with other donors and agencies. With UNAIDS, the Bank will bring together key sectors of governments and many development partners to forge strategic country and regional responses to HIV/AIDS.

•   •   •

Conclusion

Asia will determine the future of the global HIV/AIDS pandemic. Fortunately, many countries have already begun to fight. But there is much to be done. The World Bank, in close partnership with government, civil society, and other partners can also assist in this response—at both the country and the regional levels. Working with these partners, the World Bank can play a critical role in addressing the risks associated with HIV/AIDS epidemics in the East Asia and Pacific Region to prevent the region from becoming the future epicenter of HIV/AIDS.

ANNEX 1

Classification of the Epidemic

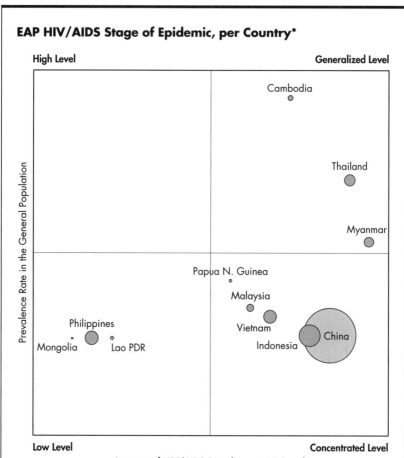

EAP HIV/AIDS Stage of Epidemic, per Country*

High Level   Generalized Level

Prevalence Rate in the General Population

Cambodia

Thailand

Myanmar

Papua N. Guinea

Malaysia

Philippines   Vietnam   China

Mongolia   Lao PDR   Indonesia

Low Level   Concentrated Level

Average of HIV/AIDS Prevalence in HRG with
Highest Prevalence Rates (Scored)

 Bubble size is proportional to population in country

*Note: (1) In Y axis, countries were scored in decreasing order according to weighted averages of the
highest HIV/AIDS prevalence rate among groups practicing high-risk behaviors (HRG); (2) Available
data from 1994 to 2003.
• **Generalized:** Greater than 1% among women attending antenatal clinics
• **Concentrated:** Greater than 5% among STD patients and other risk groups
• **Low Level:** Below 1% among STD patients and other risk groups

Country Overviews

The following country overviews provide a snapshot of HIV/AIDS data, programs, and policies in several of the countries in the EAP Region. It must be noted that there are many discrepancies in the available data. Thus in order to provide the greatest level of standardization, all data were first taken from one single source, if possible, and then supplemented with other data when available.

The primary sources of data are:

- Population numbers and prevalence data: UNAIDS Epidemiological Fact Sheets by Country (UNAIDS/WHO, 2002)

- Number of people on antiretroviral therapy: background paper from Julian Gold (Gold and Smith 2003)

- Tuberculosis data: *WHO Report 2003: Global Tuberculosis Control: Surveillance, Planning, Financing* (WHO 2003)

- Blood safety: background paper from Julian Gold (Gold and Dax 2003)

- GNI: *World Development Indicators 2001* (World Bank 2001) (http://www.worldbank.org/data/wdi2001/)

- Snapshot of selected HIV/AIDS donors[17]: Lin and Heywood 2002; Asian Development Bank (ADB); AusAID; Development Gateway; DFID; GFATM; JICA; KFW; UNAIDS; UNDP; UNICEF; USAID; World Bank; M. Morimitsu, personal communication, Japan International Corporation Agency, Tokyo, 2003; Gold and Wilson 2002

- Modes of transmission: *UNAIDS Epidemiological Fact Sheets by Country* (UNAIDS/WHO 2002)

- Injecting drug user (IDU) data: Reid and Costigan 2002

Other information was provided by numerous sources, including: USAID (http://www.usaid.gov/); NASB/MOH 2003; NASB 2002; World Bank: *World Development Indicators;* Burrows, personal communication, The Burnet Institute, Melbourne, Australia, 2003; Khorloo 2003; Reid and Costigan 2002; Feng, undated; WHO: *HIV/AIDS in Asia and the Pacific Region* (WHO 2001); GFATM applications.

CAMBODIA

HIV Epidemic Status: Generalized

Total population: 13,441,000
HIV Prevalence in Adult Population (15–49 years old) 2.7% (160,000/6,314,000)
HIV Prevalence in Female Sex Workers 26.3–31%
HIV Prevalence in Injecting Drug Users . . . . Unknown
HIV Prevalence in Women in Antenatal Clinics 0.6–5.7%
HIV Prevalence in Male STI Patients (urban) 8.5%
Number of People on Antiretroviral Therapy 750
Estimated Incidence of TB (all cases/100,000 pop) 585
Estimated Adult Cases of TB that Are HIV+ (%) 20
Estimated Multidrug Resistance (new cases) 4.2
Per Capita Gross National Income (US$, 2000) 270

Modes of Transmission in Reported HIV/AIDS Cases (%)
• Unknown 96.1
• Hetero 3.9

World Bank Projects with HIV Components
• **1997:** Disease Control and Health Development Project, 30.4 million total, 6.1 million HIV
• **2002:** Health Sector Support Project, 27.0 million total, 2.0 million HIV

Snapshot of Selected Other Donors (U.S. millions)
• USAID: Reduced transmission of STIs and HIV/AIDS in high-risk populations (1998–2002): *2.05 (2000) / 2.50 (2001)*
• JICA: Equipment Supply Program for AIDS Control and Blood Tests (2000): *0.16*
• DFID: UNAIDS (2001–02): *0.10*
• DFID: Enhancing the response to HIV/AIDS (2001–06): *14.05*
• UNDP: Multisectoral assistance to the HIV/AIDS Program in Cambodia (1996–2000): *0.95*
• ADB: Technical assistance to Cambodia for capacity building for HIV/AIDS prevention and control (2001–02): *0.07*
• French Cooperation: Technical assistance to MOH and support for access to treatment (2000–05): *1.25*

Global Fund (U.S. millions)
• Partnerships for going to scale with proven interventions for HIV/AIDS, TB, and malaria: *30.8*

Blood Safety
• **Policy:** Since 1994. 2000—National blood policy. This policy confirms that the MOH has ultimate responsibility for the management of the National Blood Transfusion Service (NBTS).
• **Strategic Plan:** In draft for 2003–07. Financed by MOH. Aims are to ensure sustainable self-sufficiency in safe blood and blood products.
• **Present Structure:** Hospital based with a national center National Blood Transfusion Committee (NBTC).
• **Statistics:** 2 donations per 1,000 population; 70% replacement donors; 27% external blood donors; through mobile collection teams; 3% spontaneous regular donors. Quality assessment program for HIV testing from Pasteur Institute. Clinical guidelines available. 90% of blood transfusions are whole blood transfusions.

The National Center for HIV/AIDS, Dermatology, and STD (NCHADS) is situated within the Health Ministry; it is the older of two AIDS bodies that has responsibility for a health response to AIDS. The National AIDS Authority (NAA) has evolved into a cross-cutting body promoting action against AIDS across governments.

MYANMAR

HIV Epidemic Status: Generalized

Total population: 48,364,000

HIV Prevalence in Adult Population (15–49 years old) . . . . Unknown
HIV Prevalence in Female Sex Workers. 26–50%
HIV Prevalence in Injecting Drug Users 37.1–63%
HIV Prevalence in Women in Antenatal Clinics 0.0–5.3%
HIV Prevalence in Male STI Patients (urban) 12.1–13.0%
Number of People on Antiretroviral Therapy . . . . Unknown
Estimated Incidence of TB (all cases/100,000 pop) 162
Estimated Adult Cases of TB that Are HIV+ (%) 11
Estimated Multidrug Resistance (new cases) 1.5
Per Capita Gross National Income (US$, 2000) 390

Modes of Transmission in Reported HIV/AIDS Cases (%)
- Hetero 57.0
- IDU 22.1
- Unknown 13.5
- Blood 4.4
- Perinatal. 1.8
- Homo/Bi 1.2

Snapshot of Selected Other Donors (U.S. millions)
- AusAID: UNICEF: Mekong Subregional HIV/AIDS Program (1999–2002): *0.77*
- AusAID: WVA: Eastern Shan State HIV/AIDS Project (1998–2002): *0.19*
- AusAID: WVA: Southern Myanmar HIV/AIDS Project (1998–2002): *0.19*
- DFID: Community action for HIV/AIDS care and support in the Mekong Subregion (2001–04): *0.34*
- JICA: Equipment Supply Program for AIDS Control and Blood Tests (2000–02): *0.55*

Global Fund (U.S. millions)
- Strengthening of Prevention and Control Program on HIV/AIDS and Malaria: *54.3*

Injecting Drug Use
- Estimated Number of IDUs: 150,000–250,000
- Status of Interventions for IDUs: No substitution therapy; no needle exchange program

THAILAND

HIV Epidemic Status: Generalized

Total population: 63,584,000
HIV Prevalence in Adult Population (15–49 years old) 1.8% (650,000/36,600,000)
HIV Prevalence in Female Sex Workers. 6.7–10.5%
HIV Prevalence in Injecting Drug Users 39.6–50%
HIV Prevalence in Women in Antenatal Clinics. 0.4–5.3%
HIV Prevalence in Male STI Patients (urban) 2.5%
Number of People on Antiretroviral Therapy. 20,000
Estimated Incidence of TB (all cases/100,000 pop) 135
Estimated Adult Cases of TB that Are HIV+ (%) 12
Estimated Multidrug Resistance (new cases) 2.1
Per Capita Gross National Income (US$, 2000) 2,020

Modes of Transmission in Reported HIV/AIDS Cases (%)
• Hetero 82.4
• Unknown 7.1
• IDU 4.8
• Perinatal. 4.6
• Homo/Bi 1.1

World Bank Projects with HIV Components
• **1998:** Social Investment Project, 300 million total, 2.6 million HIV

Snapshot of Selected Other Donors (U.S. millions)
• AusAID: Ambulatory Care Project (2000–01): *0.51*
• JICA: Project for Model Development of Comprehensive HIV/AIDS Prevention and Care (1998–2003): *4.72*
• JICA: Equipment Supply Program for AIDS Control and Blood Tests (2002): *0.03*
• UNDP: HIV/AIDS prevention and care (1994–2000): *0.80*
• UNDP: Prevention and control of AIDS in Thailand (1989–2000): *0.89*

Global Fund (U.S. millions)
• Strengthening national prevention and care programs on HIV/AIDS, tuberculosis, and malaria in Thailand: *109.5*
• National prevention and control program of HIV/AIDS and malaria in Thailand: *81.3*
• Preventing HIV/AIDS and increasing care and support for injection drug users in Thailand: *1.37*

Injecting Drug Use
• Estimated Number of IDUs: Currently unknown (in 1994, 100,000–250,000)
• Status of Interventions for IDUs: First country to introduce widespread use of methadone as substitution therapy

CHINA

HIV Epidemic Status: Concentrated

Total population: 1,284,972,000
HIV Prevalence in Adult Population (15–49 years old) 0.1% (850,000/726,031,000)
HIV Prevalence in Female Sex Workers 0–10.3%
HIV Prevalence in Injecting Drug Users. 0–80%
HIV Prevalence in Women in Antenatal Clinics 0–0.5%
HIV Prevalence in Male STI Patients (urban) 0–1.3%
Number of People on Antiretroviral Therapy 3,000
Estimated Incidence of TB (all cases/100,000 pop) 113
Estimated Adult Cases of TB that Are HIV+ (%). 0.4
Estimated Multidrug Resistance (new cases) 5.3
Per Capita Gross National Income (US$, 2000). 840

Modes of Transmission in Reported HIV/AIDS Cases (%)
- IDU 38.4
- Unknown 32.9
- Hetero 23.0
- Blood 4.0
- Homo/Bi 1.4
- Perinatal 0.4

World Bank Projects with HIV Components
- **1996:** Disease Prevention Project, 100 million total, 4.95 million HIV
- **1999:** Health Nine Project, 60 million total, 25.6 million HIV
- **2002:** Tuberculosis Control Project, 104 million total, 0.1 million HIV

Snapshot of Selected Other Donors (U.S. millions)
- AusAID: HIV/AIDS Prevention and Care Project (2002–07): *7.54*
- DFID: HIV/AIDS Economic Impact Study (2001–02): *0.18*
- DFID: HIV/AIDS Education Project (2001–06): *0.22*
- DFID: Support for HIV/AIDS education for young people (2001–06): *21.87*
- UNDP: Multisector approaches for HIV/AIDS control and prevention in China (1997–2000): *1.90*

Global Fund (U.S. millions)
- China Comprehensive AIDS Response: *97.9*

Blood Safety
- **Policy:** BTS are nonprofit organizations; 1984 nonremunerated, voluntary donor policy became law in 1998.
- **Strategic Plan:** MOH issued temporary administrative measures in 1998. Standards for BTS are under development.
- **Present Structure:** One BTS per province; one central BTS for each municipality.
- **Statistics:** 53% volunteer donors.

Injecting Drug Use
- Estimated Number of IDUs: 3.5 million
- Status of Interventions for IDUs: Methadone maintenance and needle/syringe social marketing are now being piloted.

In May 2001, the State Council issued a 5-year action plan (2001–05), with two priority action areas: (a) health education to develop a basic understanding of HIV prevention in the general population and (b) behavioral interventions among groups that practice high-risk behaviors.

INDONESIA

HIV Epidemic Status: Concentrated

Total population: 214,840,000
HIV Prevalence in Adult Population (15–49 years old) 0.1% (120,000/118,000)
HIV Prevalence in Female Sex Workers 2.0–27%
HIV Prevalence in Injecting Drug Users 19–48%
HIV Prevalence in Women in Antenatal Clinics 0.0%
HIV Prevalence in Male STI Patients (urban) . . . . Unknown
Number of People on Antiretroviral Therapy . . . . Unknown
Estimated Incidence of TB (all cases/100,000 pop) 271
Estimated Adult Cases of TB that Are HIV+ (%) 0.3
Estimated Multidrug Resistance (new cases) 0.7
Per Capita Gross National Income (US$, 2000) 580

Modes of Transmission in Reported HIV/AIDS Cases (%)
- Hetero 55.5
- IDU 18.7
- Homo/Bi 14.2
- Unknown 9.6
- Perinatal 1.4
- Blood 0.6

World Bank Projects with HIV Components
- 1996: HIV/AIDS and STD Prevention and Management Project, 24.8 million total, 24.8 million for HIV (project was closed in 1999, disbursing $4.52 million of the $24.8 million)
- 1998: Safe Motherhood Project, 42.5 million total, 0.2 million HIV

Snapshot of Selected Other Donors (U.S. millions)
- AusAID: HIV/AIDS Prevention and Care Project–Phase 1 (1998–2002): *21.0*
- AusAID: HIV/AIDS Prevention and Care Project–Phase 2 (2002–07): *30.0*
- KFW: HIV/AIDS Prevention and Family Planning (2000–03): *9.42*
- UNDP: Strengthening GOI/NGO Capacity and Partnership for HIV/AIDS Program implementation (1997–2000): *0.88*

Global Fund (U.S. millions)
- Strengthening directly observed treatment (short course) (DOTS) expansion in Indonesia (HIV/AIDS): *15.96*

Blood Safety
- **Policy:** Has a blood policy but not implemented.
- **Strategic Plan:** Two systems—a government and a hospital-based system.
- **Present Structure:** Province based over the last 3 years.
- **Statistics:** Very little blood collected for the large population.

Injecting Drug Use
- Estimated Number of IDUs: 150,000
- Status of Interventions for IDUs: Pilot project on substitution therapy; pilot project on needle exchange and outreach

MALAYSIA

HIV Epidemic Status: Concentrated

Total population: 22,633,000

HIV Prevalence in Adult Population (15–49 years old) 0.4% (41,000/11,800,000)
HIV Prevalence in Female Sex Workers 2.05–6.3%
HIV Prevalence in Injecting Drug Users. 16.8%
HIV Prevalence in Women in Antenatal Clinics 0.0–0.7%
HIV Prevalence in Male STI Patients (urban) 4.2%
Number of People on Antiretroviral Therapy . . . . <100
Per Capita Gross National Income (US$, 2000). 3,250

In 2003, there were 27,119 cases of TB in Malaysia, with a rate of 120/100,000.

Modes of Transmission in Reported HIV/AIDS Cases (%)
- IDU 54.7
- Hetero 21.2
- Unknown 21.1
- Homo/Bi 1.6
- Perinatal. 1.1
- Blood 0.3

World Bank Projects with HIV Components
- 1994: Health, 50.0 million total, 16.0 million HIV

Snapshot of Selected Other Donors (U.S. millions)
- JICA: Equipment Supply Program for AIDS Control and Blood Tests (2000): 0.22

Blood Safety
- **Policy:** Detailed policy since ~1999.
- **Strategic Plan:** Plan documented by MOH; BTS funded by MOH; move toward centralizing BTSs; central blood service seeking Good Manufacturing Practice (GMP) accreditation.
- **Present Structure:** MOH advised by a Transfusion Committee; BTS often hospital-based central services seeking GMP accreditation.

PAPUA NEW GUINEA

HIV Epidemic Status: Concentrated

Total population: 4,920,000
HIV Prevalence in Adult Population (15–49 years old) 0.7% (16,000/2,491,000)
HIV Prevalence in Female Sex Workers 16%
HIV Prevalence in Injecting Drug Users . . . . Unknown
HIV Prevalence in Women in Antenatal Clinics 0–0.2%
HIV Prevalence in Male STI Patients (urban) 7.0%
Number of People on Antiretroviral Therapy . . . . <100
Per Capita Gross National Income (US$, 2000) 670

The national incidence of TB has risen from 0.8 per 1,000 in 1974 to 10.7 per 1,000 in 1984 to 51 per 1,000 in 1999. In 2003, there were 11,602 cases, with a rate of 236/100,000.

Modes of Transmission in Reported HIV/AIDS Cases (%)
- Unknown 76.1
- Hetero 21.5
- Perinatal 1.5
- Homo/Bi 0.6
- Blood 0.3

World Bank Projects with HIV Components
- 1993: Population and family planning, 6.9 million total, 0.66 million HIV

Snapshot of Selected Other Donors (U.S. millions)
- AusAID (2000–05): *30.78*

Blood Safety
- **Policy:** Papua New Guinea Red Cross does not have a policy document.
- **Strategic Plan:** BTS operates under a Memorandum of Understanding (MOU) between the Department of Health (DOH) and Red Cross. Future plan: Government to rebuild BTS headquarters (HQ) laboratory (AusAID funding) and retrain all staff (AusAID funding). BTS: Phenotyping panel cell preparation. Plasmapheresis unit establishment. Red Cross: Withdrawal from BTS management after termination of MOU with DOH in 2003 and concentrate on developing donor recruitment only.
- **Present Structure:** MOU outlines that DOH is responsible for finance, buildings, staff, and equipment and materials. Most of the guidelines are incorporated in the Standard Operating Procedure (SOP) manual and DOH/Red Cross MOU. MOU terminates in 2003. Quality control exists. Internal controls at each blood bank.
- **Statistics:** 50% blood donation voluntary, 49% family/replacement, <1% voluntary regular blood donors. Each hospital collects blood for its own use mainly as red cell concentrate and whole blood. Only BTS HQ produces fresh-frozen plasma, cryoprecipitate, and platelet concentrates.

2003: Legislation was designed that could improve the management of AIDS. The proposal includes human rights, proscribes national policy and practice on HIV testing and medical management, and provides voluntary counseling and testing.

VIETNAM

HIV Epidemic Status: Concentrated

Total population: 79,175,000
HIV Prevalence in Adult Population (15–49 years old) 0.3% (130,000/43,300,000)
HIV Prevalence in Female Sex Workers 4.2–6.0%
HIV Prevalence in Injecting Drug Users 26.8–30.4%
HIV Prevalence in Women in Antenatal Clinics 0.0–0.4%
HIV Prevalence in Male STI Patients (urban) 2.0–3.2%
Number of People on Antiretroviral Therapy . . . . Approx. 50 in pilot study
Estimated Incidence of TB (all cases/100,000 pop) 179
Estimated Adult Cases of TB that Are HIV+ (%) 1.4
Estimated Multidrug Resistance (new cases) 2.3
Per Capita Gross National Income (US$, 2000) 390

Modes of Transmission in Reported HIV/AIDS Cases (%)
- Unknown 52.4
- IDU 38.2
- Hetero 8.6
- Perinatal 0.8

World Bank Projects with HIV Components
- **2002:** Regional Blood Transfusion Centers Project, 38.2 million total, 38.2 million HIV

Snapshot of Selected Other Donors (U.S. millions)
- AusAID: HIV/AIDS Capacity Building Project (2002–04): *0.82*
- AusAID: UNDP HIV/AIDS Youth Awareness Project (2002–05): *0.71*
- AusAID: Care: NOVA2000: Confronting HIV/AIDS, project-NGO window (2000–03): *0.35*
- AusAID: Participatory HIV/AIDS prevention (1998–2001): *0.57*
- AusAID: UNDP/HIV/AIDS: Awareness raising for youth, cofinancing (2000–03): *1.14*
- UNDP: HIV/AIDS capacity building (1999–2001): *0.75*
- UNDP: HIV/AIDS, environment, and youth (1999–2001): *0.63*
- UNDP: Strengthening the capacity for coordination, management, and planning of HIV/AIDS in Vietnam (1994–2000): *1.04*
- DFID: HIV/AIDS control (2001–02): *24.59*

Global Fund (U.S. millions)
- Strengthening care, counseling, support to people living with HIV/AIDS (PLWHAs), and related community-based activities: *12.00*

Blood Safety
- The Regulation for Blood Transfusion issues in 1992 established standards and guidelines for blood safety. By 2000, the blood safety program had reached its objective of 100% blood units screened for HIV. Strategy for blood collection was recently shifted from collecting at district health facilities to provincial or regional facilities.

Injecting Drug Use
- Estimated Number of IDUs: 69,000 (1997)

LAO PDR

HIV Epidemic Status: Low Level

Total population: 5,403,000
HIV Prevalence in Adult Population (15–49 years old) . . . . <0.1% (1,300/2,500,000)
HIV Prevalence in Female Sex Workers 1.0%
HIV Prevalence in Injecting Drug Users 2.0%
HIV Prevalence in Women in Antenatal Clinics 0.0%
HIV Prevalence in Male STI Patients (urban) . . . . Unknown
Number of People on Antiretroviral Therapy . . . . Unknown
Per Capita Gross National Income (US$, 2000) 290

The national incidence of TB has risen from 0.8 per 1,000 in 1974 to 10.7 per 1,000 in 1984 to 51 per 1,000 in 1999. In 2003, there were 8,512 cases in Lao PDR with a rate of 158/100,000.

Modes of Transmission in Reported HIV/AIDS Cases (%)
- Unknown 97.7
- Perinatal 2.3

Snapshot of Selected Other Donors (U.S. millions)
- AusAID: Mekong Subregional HIV/AIDS Care and Support Project (2000–02): *0.52*
- USAID: HIV/AIDS (2002–06): *1.00* (2002)–*1.00* (2003)
- JICA: Equipment Supply Program for AIDS Control and Blood Tests (2000): *0.17*
- UNDP: Lao PDR HIV/AIDS (1998–2000): *0.27*

Global Fund (U.S. millions)
- Prevention and control of HIV/AIDS/STI, TB, and malaria in the Lao PDR: *3.4*

Blood Safety
- **Policy:** In 1991 the MOH transferred BTS to the Lao Red Cross. Quality system is in place but not formal.
- **Strategic Plan:** Reconsidering the organization system of the BTS and its tasks.
- **Present Structure:** NBTC plus eight provinces exist.
- **Statistics:** 80% blood is collected from mobile sessions, ~11,000 blood units are annually supplied, 63% is collected from voluntary donors.

Lao PDR developed a National Strategic Plan (NSP) on HIV/AIDS/STD for 2002–05. Main issues declared as priorities included surveillance, STD prevention and treatment, and prevention of HIV among youth, mobile populations, and service women.

MONGOLIA

HIV Epidemic Status: Low Level

Total population: 2,559,000
HIV Prevalence in Adult Population (15–49 years old) . . . . <0.1% (<100/1,400,000)
HIV Prevalence in Female Sex Workers . . . . Unknown
HIV Prevalence in Injecting Drug Users . . . . No reported cases
HIV Prevalence in Women in Antenatal Clinics . . . . Unknown
HIV Prevalence in Male STI Patients (urban) 0.0%
Number of People on Antiretroviral Therapy . . . . Unknown
Per Capita Gross National Income (US$, 2000) 390

In 2003, there were 4,969 TB cases in Mongolia with a rate of 194/100,000.

Modes of Transmission in Reported HIV/AIDS Cases (%)
• Hetero 50
• Homo/Bi 50

Snapshot of Selected Other Donors (U.S. millions)
• AusAID: STI/HIV education (UNDP), cofinancing (2000–02): *249.05*
• UNDP: HIV/AIDS/STDs in Mongolia (1997–2000): *0.30*

Global Fund (U.S. millions)
• Strengthening national prevention and care programs on HIV/AIDS in Mongolia: *3.0*

Blood Safety
• **Policy:** 2000 National Blood Policy exists.
• **Strategic Plan:** Central BTS; 25 centers in the country.
• **Present Structure:** Areas of the country are very remote and not well planned for.
• **Statistics:** Replacement donation. Need for training, quality management, and quality assurance on all levels. Number of transfusions difficult to document.

PHILIPPINES

HIV Epidemic Status: Low Level

Total population: 77,131,000

HIV Prevalence in Adult Population (15–49 years old). . . . . . <0.1% (9,400/39,600,000)
HIV Prevalence in Female Sex Workers 0.3%
HIV Prevalence in Injecting Drug Users 1.0%
HIV Prevalence in Women in Antenatal Clinics . . . . Unknown
HIV Prevalence in Male STI Patients (urban). 0.0%
Number of People on Antiretroviral Therapy . . . . <200
Estimated Incidence of TB (all cases/100,000 pop) 297
Estimated Adult Cases of TB that Are HIV + (%) 0.4
Estimated Multidrug Resistance (new cases). 3.2
Per Capita Gross National Income (US$, 2000) 1,020

Modes of Transmission in Reported HIV/AIDS Cases (%)
- Hetero 56.0
- Homo/Bi 35.0
- Unknown 4.0
- Perinatal. 2.0
- Blood 2.0
- IDU 1.0

Snapshot of Selected Other Donors (U.S. millions)
- USAID: The threat of HIV/AIDS and selected infectious diseases is reduced (1994–2004): *4.40* (2000)
- USAID: The threat of HIV/AIDS and selected infectious diseases is reduced (1992–2004): *3.50* (2001)
- JICA: Project for Prevention and Control of AIDS (1996–2001): *7.44*
- JICA: Equipment Supply Program for AIDS Control and Blood Tests (1996–98, 2000): *1.11*
- UNDP: Promoting multisectoral and community-based approaches to HIV prevention and care in the Philippines (2000): *0.26*
- UNDP: Increasing awareness and understanding of the development implications of HIV/AIDS (2000): *0.15*

Global Fund (U.S. millions)
- Accelerating STI and HIV/AIDS prevention through intensified delivery of services to vulnerable groups and people living with HIV/AIDS in strategic areas in the Philippines: *5.5*

Blood Safety
- **Policy:** Policies and guidelines are well developed but not followed. 1994—National Blood Services Act.
- **Present Structure:** National Center with regional directors. National Reference Laboratory is designated.

Injecting Drug Use
- Estimated Number of IDUs: 10,000
- Status of Interventions for IDUs: No substitution therapy; no needle exchange program

The AIDS Prevention and Control Act was signed into law in February 1998. It created a legal and policy environment to prevent new infections and protect the human rights and civil liberties of people living with HIV/AIDS.

Snapshot of Estimated Number and Risk Behaviors of Injecting Drug Users and Commercial Sex Workers in the <u>EAP Region</u>

The information in both of these tables was compiled using data from numerous sources and is therefore not standardized. This is only to be used as an example of the variety and size of risk behaviors in the region.

Country	Estimated number of IDUs	Risk behaviors	Drug used	HIV prevalence among IDUs
Generalized				
Cambodia	Unknown	Little evidence of injecting drug use	Heroin, blackwater opium	Unknown
Myanmar	150,000–250,000	Widespread high-risk behaviors in "shooting galleries," sharing of needles and syringes	Heroin	37.1–63%, in some states as high as 90%, among the highest in the world
Thailand	Unknown (in 1994; 100,000–250,000)	Frequency of injecting, widespread sharing of needles	Heroin, opium, methamphetamines	39.6–50% (2000/2001)
Concentrated				
China	3.5 million	Sharing of needles and syringes, mixing heroin with blood and passing it around to other drug users	Heroin, methamphetamine, diazepam mixed with heroin, cooked opium juice, ketamine	0–20.5% (2000); up to 80% according to the region
Indonesia	150,000	Sharing of injecting equipment, inadequate or no cleaning of the equipment	Heroin, methamphetamine, benzodiazapines	19–48% (2001/2002)

Malaysia	200,000	Sharing of injecting equipment, inadequate cleaning of the equipment, professional injectors using the same unsterile injecting equipment with multiple customers	Heroin	16.8% (1996), up to 76.3%
Vietnam	69,000	Sharing of injecting equipment, condom use among IDUs low	Heroin, blackwater opium, morphine, pethidine, promethazine, diazepam, phenobarbital	26.8–30.4% (2003), up to 89.9%
Low level				
Lao PDR	Unknown, but considered low	—	Blackwater opium, amphetamines, some heroin	2%
Mongolia	No official estimates	Growing tendency toward use of drugs for recreational purposes, clear signs of linkages between IDUs and CSWs	Cannabis, diazepam, dimedrol	No reported cases
Philippines	10,000	Sharing of needles and syringes	Nubain, drug cocktails	1%, but WHO estimates to be higher

Blank cells: Information not available.

Source: *Epidemiological Fact Sheets by Country–2002 Updates* (UNAIDS/WHO 2002); *Report on the Global HIV/AIDS Epidemic* (UNAIDS 2002); Reid and Costigan 2002; Khorloo 2003; Feng, undated; NASB/MOH 2003; NASB 2002; World Bank 2003; Pisani and others 2003.

Country	Estimated number of CSWs	Risk behaviors	Risk clients	HIV prevalence
Generalized				
Cambodia	12,290 (high est.)	Unprotected sexual intercourse, partner exchange pattern is one of the highest in the region	Age group (15–49), Average rate (33.0); Mean number of clients in the previous night was 3.2 per CSW	26.3–31% (2001/02)
Myanmar	—	Link between IDUs and CSWs, unsafe sexual practices	Age group (18–49), rate (7.77)	26–50% (2000)
Thailand	—	—	The % of adult men visiting CSWs has fallen from almost 25% to roughly 10%	6.7% (major urban), 10.5% (outside major urban) (2000)
Concentrated				
China	More than 3 million	Increasing involvement of female IDUs in prostitution, very large proportion of female sex workers never use condoms (more than 49%)	—	0–10.3% (major urban), 0–2.9% (outside major urban) (2000)
Indonesia	Between 200,000 and 270,000	Low use of condoms in commercial encounters: virtually unchanged since surveillance began	About 32,000 clients infected with HIV, average number of clients per week (7.8). Sailors and truckers report much higher level of contact with CSWs than any other groups	2.0–27% (2002)

Country				
Malaysia	50,000		—	6.3% (major urban), 2.05% (outside major urban) (1996)
Papua New Guinea	—	Low level of condom use in casual partnership	—	16% (2002)
Vietnam	—	Prevalence of IDU ranges from 10% to 50%, consistent use of condoms is lowest in Ho Chi Minh City (avg. 40%)	Average number of clients per CSW (3–5 per week) Frequency of contact is around 60 times/month/SW	4.2–6.0% (2002/03)
Low level				
Lao PDR[a]	Average number of service women : 15–19 (35.7), 20–24 (40.3), 25–29 (16.7), ≥30 (7.4)	Increasing number of sex workers, cross-border population movement	About a third of truck drivers and a quarter of police reported paying for sex, 32% of truck drivers and 24% of police reported 3 or more partners in the past year	1.0% (2000)
Mongolia	—	—	—	—
Philippines	—	—	Average low number of clients (2.2–3.5 per week, 1999)	0.3% (1994)

a. Formal sex work is rare in Lao PDR, and prostitution is illegal. However, 68% of service women reported having either a commercial or nonregular sex partner in the past year.

Blank cells: Information not available.

Source: *Epidemiological Fact Sheets by Country—2002 Updates* (UNAIDS/WHO 2002); *Report on the Global HIV/AIDS Epidemic* (UNAIDS 2002); NASB/MOH 2003; NASB 2002; World Bank 2003; Pisani and others 2003.

ANNEX 4

Infectious Disease Epidemiology

All socioeconomic models of the impact of HIV/AIDS depend on epidemiological predictions on the future course of the epidemic. Many economic models rely on simplistic assumptions that other parts of the world will follow the trajectory of Sub-Saharan Africa. This analogy reflects a profound misunderstanding of the epidemiology of HIV. To understand this one must develop a theoretical model of the growth of infectious diseases.

Infectious diseases do not grow indefinitely—there must be some natural limit. In fact, when one views an epidemic over time, it has an initial phase of growth and then it tapers off and reaches a steady state before it eventually disappears. The classic case of this type of infection is influenza or SARS. HIV/AIDS is similar, but the process is much slower because of the long interval between infection with HIV and the development of AIDS. In addition, there is a long period of infectiousness, often years, which makes it very different from classical infectious diseases such as influenza.

The figure on page 72 shows the course of an HIV/AIDS infection in a population.[18] The key to understanding the dynamics of an infectious disease is the reproductive rate (R_0) common to all organisms.

As can be seen, in the initial period of $R_0 > 1$, the prevalence increases exponentially. However, as the number of people susceptible to the disease are "used up" by the epidemic, the reproductive rate begins to fall. If no new susceptible groups enter the population, then the infection will fade away. Given the long duration of HIV/AIDS, there is continuing growth in new susceptible populations, making extinction unlikely.

Course of an HIV/AIDS Infection

A. Reproductive Rates for an HIV/AIDS Epidemic

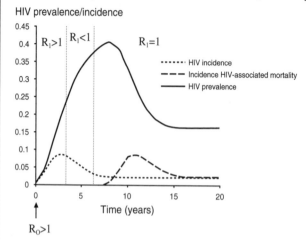

HIV prevalence/incidence

$R_1 > 1$ $R_1 < 1$ $R_1 = 1$

······ HIV incidence
― ― ― Incidence HIV-associated mortality
――― HIV prevalence

Time (years)

$R_0 > 1$

B. Stages of an HIV/AIDS Epidemic

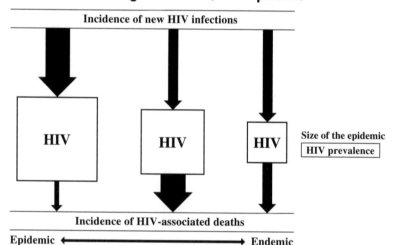

Incidence of new HIV infections

HIV   HIV   HIV   Size of the epidemic
                                        HIV prevalence

Incidence of HIV-associated deaths

Epidemic ←――――――――――――→ Endemic

Note: The relationship between the effective reproductive rate R, the incidence of HIV infections, and HIV prevalence is shown in (**A**). For simplicity, it is assumed that all incident cases of HIV die 8 years after infection. In this simple case, the incidence of AIDS deaths replicates HIV incidence. On entry to the population, the effective reproductive rate equals the basis reproductive rate and must be greater than 1 for an epidemic to occur. As the presence of infection increases, the effective reproductive rate decreases as contacts are made with those already infected. The epidemic continues to grow even when each new case generates fewer than one more case, because infections are still occurring. Incidence decreases before prevalence; only when deaths remove those infected from population will prevalence decrease. The relationship between incident HIV infections and incident HIV-associated mortality is illustrated in (**B**). When incident infections match incident deaths, the epidemic will have reached an endemic steady state. Here the average effective reproductive rate must be 1 if the prevalence is to remain constant.

Source: Garnett 1998.

What determines the value of R_0?

$R_0 = \beta c D$

where

    β = the likelihood of transmission when a contact is made between an infected and susceptible;
    c = the rate of contact in the population; and
    D = the duration of infectiousness.

Understanding these three simple terms is the key to understanding the epidemic. β represents the transmission probability. In the case of HIV/AIDS, this is the probability that HIV will be spread between two individuals based on their contact. For sexual contact this is the probability of transmission during the sex act, which is estimated to be quite low (0.001). Concurrent STIs increase β 50- to 300-fold. The β for transmission by sharing contaminated needles is significantly higher.

The other key variable is c, the pattern of contacts. This simple concept is very complex because it depends on the overall sexual networks. There has been a large growth of sexual behavioral studies. Unfortunately, there has been limited growth in Asia and much more work is needed to more fully understand the sexual networks in Asia. One of the key differences compared with North America and Western Europe is the common use of commercial sex workers in Asian countries by men from a wide range of age groups and social classes. In Thailand, before HIV/AIDS, it was estimated that more than a quarter of the population visited sex workers.

The final variable is D, the duration of effectiveness, which would be affected by treatment. This simple model can be increased in almost infinite complexity by adding subpopulations with different risk behavior and different mixing patterns with other subpopulations. As the model increases in complexity, more parameter estimates are needed.

These models play a key role in understanding epidemics. Economic models are only as good as the epidemiological-demographic projections. The models are dynamic and a country's position on the epidemic curve will determine the interventions needed and their relative cost-effectiveness. It is important to emphasize that the cost-effectiveness of interventions changes depending on the state of the epidemic. Therefore, these models are particularly useful for modeling interventions and comparing relative cost-effectiveness. They can be a useful tool for program planning and for determining coverage targets needed to alter the course of the epidemic. They are also an important tool in predicting the trajectory of the HIV epidemic. There is an urgent need to standardize these models and improve data collection for parameters.

Epidemiological Projections of HIV/AIDS in East Asia

Although there are limited data, many observers have made predictions concerning the course of the EAP epidemic. These range from rates similar to Sub-Saharan Africa to a prediction that most Asian epidemics will never reach 1 percent prevalence.

The predictions of large-scale growth of Asian epidemics are based on the experience of Sub-Saharan Africa, where concentrated epidemics began in groups practicing high-risk behavior, and then HIV spread to the general population. Under this scenario, Asia is at great risk for becoming the epicenter of the HIV epidemic in the next decade.

This was the approach adopted by the U.S. Central Intelligence Agency[19] in its scenario planning and reinforced by Eberstadt's model,[20] which presumes the epidemic will become a sexually transmitted disease in the general population. According to Eberstadt, Eurasia (considered to be the continent of Asia, plus Russia) could soon house the largest number of AIDS victims, driven by the spread of HIV in China, India, and Russia. Even under the assumption of a mild epidemic, Eberstadt suggests that the total number of HIV cases in China, India, and Russia from 2000 through 2025 would equal 66 million. With high rates, China would alone account for 70 million new cases.

Eberstadt predicts that even a mild epidemic would have dire economic effects leading to a decrease in economic growth by half.

There is a countervailing view from some epidemiologists that Asian epidemics are constrained by low-sexual-risk behavior in the general population (Chin 2003).[21] Some analysts believe that the Asian HIV epidemics will

Projections Based on the Eberstadt Model for China for 2025

China	Mild epidemic (1.5%)	Intermediate epidemic (3.5%)	Severe epidemic (5%)
Cumulative new HIV cases	32 million	70 million	100 million
Cumulative AIDS deaths	19 million	40 million	58 million

never become generalized sexual epidemics similar to Sub-Saharan Africa. According to them, there are not multiple, overlapping partners and high rates of sexually transmitted diseases that drive the African epidemics. They believe that because risk behavior in the general population is low in Asia, HIV will not become a sexually transmitted disease and spread rapidly through the general, heterosexual population. Under the scenario of low-risk behavior in the general population, they predict that concentrated epidemics will remain concentrated and they will not spread to the general population.

Such views suggest that the potential for growth in the concentrated epidemics in the region (China, Indonesia, Vietnam, and Malaysia) is low because of the lower rate of high-risk sexual behavior in the general population and the low underlying prevalence of sexually transmitted diseases. Even repeating the pattern of growth similar to Thailand and Cambodia is unlikely for these countries because of the lower level of commercial sex work with fewer men visiting CSWs and less often. According to this theory, Asian epidemics are fundamentally different from the epidemics in Sub-Saharan Africa and none will become generalized epidemics in the heterosexual population. There is one country, Papua New Guinea, where the preconditions exist for the epidemic to follow a trajectory similar to Sub-Saharan Africa.

USAID, intrigued by this hypothesis for HIV in Asia, commissioned a consortium led by Tim Brown and Wiwat Peerapatinapokin from the East-West Center to develop a transmission dynamic model of HIV/AIDS that would attempt to understand the dynamics of HIV/AIDS in Asia. The Asian Epidemic Model (AEM) has been used extensively in Thailand and Cambodia (Cambodia Working Group on HIV/AIDS Projection 2002; Thai Working Group on HIV/AIDS Projections 2001). The model captures the interaction between groups, including CSWs, their clients, IDUs, and the general population. The model requires extensive data, and Thailand is one of the few countries with adequate data to test empirically the model by comparing its projections to actual prevalence data. However, the model is actually fit to the existing data.

AEM does not predict that the growth of the epidemic would be constrained. Without interventions, the epidemic in Thailand would have continued to grow toward 10 percent by 2010. What drives the growth is the high rate of high-risk behavior among the population, with over 25 percent of men reporting having sex outside of long-term partnerships.

The AEM is a sophisticated model that requires a large amount of data, not available in most countries. UNAIDS has developed a simpler model, fairly conservative in approach, for predicting the future of the epidemic. The main consideration underlying this approach is a practical understanding of the level and quality of data for HIV/AIDS at the country level. Also, the method should be able to be used by country programs using local capacity.

The estimates are usually produced through a multimethod process using local experts with locally available data supplemented by targeted survey data. The UNAIDS projections are based on determining the size of the at-risk populations, projecting growth until HIV saturates in the high-risk population, and factoring in the transmission from groups who practice high-risk behaviors to their partners.

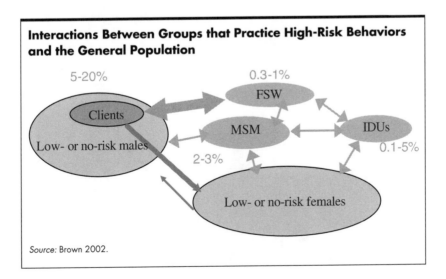

Interactions Between Groups that Practice High-Risk Behaviors and the General Population

Source: Brown 2002.

ANNEX 6

Tuberculosis

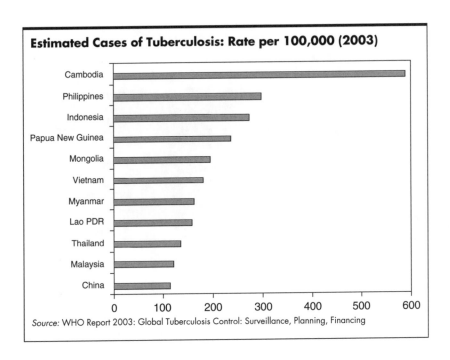

Estimated Cases of Tuberculosis: Rate per 100,000 (2003)

Cambodia	
Philippines	
Indonesia	
Papua New Guinea	
Mongolia	
Vietnam	
Myanmar	
Lao PDR	
Thailand	
Malaysia	
China	

Source: WHO Report 2003: Global Tuberculosis Control: Surveillance, Planning, Financing

ANNEX 7

Overview of Current Blood Safety Policy Status

Country	Policy	Strategic plan	Present structure	Statistics
Generalized				
Cambodia	Since 1994. 2000–National blood policy. This policy confirms the MOH has ultimate responsibility for the management of the NBTS.	In draft for 2003–07. Financed by MOH. Aims are to ensure sustainable self-sufficiency in safe blood and blood products.	Hospital-based with a national center (NBTC)	2 donations per 1,000 population. 70% replacement donors. 27% external blood donors through mobile collection teams. 3% spontaneous regular donors. Quality assessment program for HIV testing from Pasteur Institute. Clinical guidelines available. 90% of blood transfusions are whole blood transfusions. *(continued)*

Country	Policy	Strategic plan	Present structure	Statistics
Concentrated				
China	BTS are nonprofit organizations. 1984 non-remunerated, voluntary donor policy became blood donor law in 1998.	MOH issued temporary administrative measures in 1998. Standards for BTS under development.	One BTS per province. One central BTS for each municipality central BTS.	53% volunteer donors.
Indonesia	Has a blood policy but not implemented.	Two systems—a government and a hospital-based system have grown up.	Structure is province based over the last 3 years. Has resulted in fewer resources reaching the services themselves.	Very little blood collected for the very large population. Highly disorganized, under-resourced, and training is at a low level. There are exceptions such as Bali and Surabaya.
Malaysia	Detailed policy since ~1999	Plan documented by MOH. BTS funded by MOH. Move toward centralizing BTS. Central blood service seeking GMP accreditation.	MOH advised by a Transfusion Committee. BTS often hospital-based central services seeking GMP accreditation.	
Papua New Guinea	Papua New Guinea Red Cross does not have a policy document.	BTS operates under a MOU between DOH and Red Cross. Future plan: Government: rebuild BTS HQ laboratory (AusAID funding), retrain all staff (AusAID funding). BTS: pheno-typing panel cell preparation. Plasma-	MOU outlines that DOH is responsible for finance, buildings, staff, and equipment and materials. Most of the guidelines are incorporated in the SOP manual and DOH/Red Cross MOU. MOU terminates in 2003. Quality control	50% blood donation voluntary, 49% family/replacement <1% voluntary regular blood donors. Each hospital collects blood for its own use mainly as red cell concentrate and whole blood.

(continued)

Country	Policy	Strategic plan	Present structure	Statistics
		pheresis unit establishment. Red Cross: withdrawal from BTS management after termination of MOU with DOH in 2003–04 and concentrate on developing donor recruitment only.	exists. Internal controls at each blood bank.	Only BTS HQ produces fresh-frozen plasma, cryoprecipitate, and platelet concentrates (it is possible these are flown to other centers).
Low level				
Lao PDR	BTS started in 1975 under MOH. In 1991 the MOH transferred BTS to the Lao Red Cross. Quality system is in place but not formal.	Future plans will be reconsidering the organization system of the BTS and its tasks.	1995 National Blood Policy established. National Blood Transfusion Committee headed by MOH and president of Lao Red Cross set up to supervise NBP. Currently NBTC plus 8 provinces exist. Lao Red Cross governs NBC and partly governs networks in provinces. Provinces are hospital based.	Goal is 100% voluntary unpaid donors in the next few years. Mobile units are the most effective way to reach donors. 80% blood is collected from mobile sessions. Since 1995 the number of voluntary donors has increased. ~ 11,000 blood units are annually supplied, 63% is collected from voluntary donors.
Mongolia	Low level of donors—2000 National Blood Policy exists.	Central BTS. 25 centers in the country. Financed by MOH—severe financial constraints.	Areas of the country are very remote and not well planned for.	Replacement donation. Need for training, quality management, and quality assurance on all levels. Number of transfusions difficult to document.

(continued)

Country	Policy	Strategic plan	Present structure	Statistics
Philippines	Policies and guidelines are well developed but not followed. 1994–National Blood Services Act.	National policy being implemented. Commercial blood banks still operate. Financed by DOH additional funds as required.	National Center with regional directors. National Reference Laboratory is designated.	70% commercial donors (1994). 70% replacement donors (2000). 20% commercial donors (2000). National capital (2001). Voluntary donors (53%), paid (2%). 110,000 donations annually. Clinical use of blood is not under guidelines.

Source: Gold and Dax 2003.

Approved HIV-Related Projects Under the Global Fund for EAP Region

Country	Title	Round/ Status	2-year Approved	5-year Approved
Generalized				
Cambodia	Partnership for going to scale with proven interventions for HIV/AIDS, TB, and malaria	1 Approved	11,242,538	15,945,803
	Partnership for going to scale with proven interventions for HIV/AIDS, TB, and malaria	2 Approved	5,370,564	14,877,295
Myanmar	Strengthening of Prevention and Control Program on HIV/AIDS and Malaria in Myanmar	3 Approved	19,221,525	54,300,034
Thailand	Strengthening national prevention and care programs on HIV/AIDS, TB, and malaria in Thailand	1 Approved	30,933,204	109,505,316
	National prevention and control program of HIV/AIDS and malaria in Thailand	2 Approved	20,253,183	81,348,535
	Preventing HIV/AIDS and increasing care and support for injection drug users in Thailand	3 Approved	911,542	1,371,348
Concentrated				
China	China CARES (China Comprehensive AIDS RESponse)—a community-based HIV treatment, care, and prevention program in Central China	3 Approved	32,122,550	97,888,170

(continued)

Country	Title	Round/ Status	2-year Approved	5-year Approved
Indonesia	Strengthening directly observed treatment, short course expansion in Indonesia	1 Approved	6,924,971	15,960,103
Vietnam	Strengthening care, counseling, support to people living with HIV/AIDS (PLWHAs) and related community-based activities	1 Approved	7,500,000	12,000,000
Low level				
Lao PDR	Prevention and control of HIV/AIDS/sexually transmitted infections, TB, and malaria in the Lao PDR	1 Approved	1,307,664	3,407,664
Mongolia	Strengthening national prevention and care programs on HIV/AIDS in Mongolia	2 Approved	609,404	2,997,103
Multicountry Western Pacific	Pacific Islands Regional Coordinated Country Project on HIV/AIDS, TB, and Malaria (PIRCCP)	2 Approved	3,036,000	6,304,000
Philippines	Accelerating STI and HIV/AIDS prevention through intensified delivery of services to vulnerable groups and people living with HIV/AIDS in strategic areas in the Philippines	3 Approved	3,496,865	5,528,825
Total			**142,930,010**	**421,434,196**

Source: Global Fund to Fight AIDS, Tuberculosis, and Malaria, http://www.globalfundatm.org/

Notes

1. At the different stages, various risk behaviors will be the leading factors in driving the epidemic. In a majority of EAP countries such as Vietnam, China, Indonesia, and Myanmar, at the very beginning, "injecting" drug use was the driving force for the HIV epidemic, as it was responsible for the sharp increase of HIV in these countries. At least in the foreseeable future, the dual HIV epidemic among commercial sex workers and injecting drug users will be a key characteristic of HIV in the EAP Region.

2. This is the official classification of UNAIDS and the World Health Organization (WHO) (see UNAIDS/WHO 2000). It builds on the classification of the World Bank in *Confronting AIDS* (1999) with one significant difference: in the World Bank classification, the epidemic is not generalized until it reaches 5 percent prevalence in the general population. In this report, a generalized epidemic is defined as one that reaches greater than 1 percent in the general population.

3. The Pacific Island Member States include: Fiji, Kiribati, the Marshall Islands, the Federated States of Micronesia, Palau, Samoa, the Solomon Islands, Tonga, and Vanuatu.

4. Following extensive work to encourage agreement on core indicators for monitoring and evaluating HIV/AIDS programs and policies, the UNAIDS family established the Global HIV/AIDS Monitoring and Evaluation Support Team (GAMET), based at the World Bank. Other key agencies such as the Global Fund to Fight AIDS, Tuberculosis, and Malaria (GFATM), bilaterals like the United States Agency for International Development (USAID), and technical agencies such as the U.S. Centers for Disease Control and Prevention (CDC) are part of this partnership. GAMET actively works with countries and diverse donors to strengthen monitoring and evaluation

capacity at the country level, based on normative guidance from the UNAIDS Monitoring and Evaluation Reference Group. GAMET focuses, with other agencies, on helping countries to build and use monitoring and evaluation systems that will enable them to both report on progress internationally and, especially important, to identify and make tactical changes in HIV/AIDS programs and policies that improve their effectiveness.

5. Prevalence rates (determined by the number of people newly acquiring the disease plus the number of people with the disease minus those dying) can come to a steady state at differing levels. If prevalence levels off, some might believe that this means the epidemic is under control. Although this could be true (few people get the disease, few people die from the disease), the exact opposite could also be happening (large numbers of people get the disease, large numbers of people die from the disease).

6. Using the World Bank definition in *Confronting HIV/AIDS*, all of the generalized Asian epidemics would be reclassified as concentrated.

7. UNAIDS projections.

8. Much of the information in this section was drawn from the *Thailand Social Monitor* (World Bank 2000).

9. The Asian Epidemic Model predicts significant growth in the epidemic; however, other models suggest that the HIV/AIDS would decline regardless of the intervention because of saturation of high-risk populations (World Bank 1997, p. 142, Figure 3.3). Given existing data, it is difficult to determine what happened, but it is clear that there was a dramatic decline in risk behavior. This points to a need for better public health surveillance, particularly on the incidence of HIV among groups, better proxies for HIV in the general population, and more systematic information on risk behavior.

10. There are two main types of sex workers: brothel-based and "indirect." Indirect sex workers include those who work in massage parlors, restaurants, and beauty parlors, and are believed to be "higher class" (as they do not self-identify as sex workers). In addition, there are less organized forms of sex work.

11. There is great difficulty in attributing the cause of the slowing of the epidemic in Cambodia. This may be due to saturation in the epidemic. Again, greater attention is needed to monitor changes in behavior and to understand the changing incidence and death rate of HIV/AIDS.

12. This is an example of international best practice identified by UNAIDS. The study was done with officials from many ministries, including health, social affairs,

statistics, tourism, and the police. It used routine information systems from multiple sources complemented by survey data. It reduced the wide variation in estimates of injecting drug users, which ranged from 50,000 to 1 million. This is the first step in developing better estimates; the next step would be to improve routine information systems and use capture/recapture techniques. See Directorate General of Communicable Disease Control and Environmental Health 2003, and Hickman and others 2003.

13. China also has harm reduction centers that use Chinese traditional methods, in combination with short-term methadone therapy, but often with high relapse rates.

14. Ulcerative sexually transmitted diseases increase the risk of HIV transmission significantly (Chin 2003).

15. This will be supported by a grant from the GFATM. See www.gfatm.org.

16. It produces GPO-vir (a combination tablet containing nevirapine, zidovudine, and lamivudine).

17. Not all donors are included. This only serves as a snapshot of the donors in a single country.

18. The course of an HIV epidemic. The relationship between the effective reproductive rate, the incidence of HIV infections, and HIV prevalence is shown. For simplicity it is assumed that all incident cases of HIV die 8 years after infection. In this simple case, the incidence of AIDS deaths replicates HIV incidence. On entry to the population, the effective reproductive rate equals the basic reproductive rate and must be greater than 1 for an epidemic to occur. As the presence of infection increases, the effective reproductive rate decreases as contacts are made with those already infected. The epidemic continues to grow even when each new case generates fewer than one more case, because infections are still occurring. Incidence decreases before prevalence; only when deaths remove those infected from the population will prevalence decrease. The relationship between incident HIV infections and incident HIV-associated mortality is illustrated below the graph. When incident infections match incident deaths, the epidemic will have reached an endemic steady state. Here the average effective reproductive rate must be 1 if the prevalence is to remain constant.

19. NCI estimated that China currently has 1–2 million HIV cases compared with official estimates of 800,000. They expect prevalence to rise to between 1.3 and 2 percent leading to an estimate of 10–15 million HIV cases by 2010.

20. Nicholas Eberstadt, at the American Enterprise Institute, based his predictions on U.S. Bureau of the Census data analyzed using the spectrum software package

developed by the Futures Group International for USAID. His model assumes: (a) each epidemic began around 1985; (b) the median incubation period for HIV carriers between infection with HIV and the onset of AIDS is 9 years; (c) life expectancy after the onset of AIDS averages 2 years; and (d) HIV epidemics in China, India, and Russia have "standard heterosexual" distribution between sexes and age groups witnessed in other low-income countries (especially Sub-Saharan Africa) (Eberstadt 2002).

21. James Chin is formerly from the WHO Global Program for AIDS and currently a professor of epidemiology at the University of California, Berkeley.

References

Brown, T. 2002. "Understanding HIV Prevalence Differentials in Southeast Asia." East-West Center/Thai Red Cross Society. Presentation at the World Bank, Washington, D.C.

Cambodia Working Group on HIV/AIDS Projection. 2002. "Projections for HIV/AIDS in Cambodia: 2000–2010." National Center for HIV/AIDS, Dermatology and STD, Phnom Penh; Family Health International, Arlington, Va.; UCLA, Los Angeles; East-West Center, Honolulu.

Chin. 2003. "The Past, Present and Probable Future of HIV/AIDS in the East Asia and Pacific Region." World Bank, East Asia and Pacific Human Development Sector Unit, Washington, D.C.

China MOH/UNAIDS (Ministry of Health/Joint United Nations Programme on HIV/AIDS). Dec. 1, 2003. "A Joint Assessment of HIV/AIDS Prevention, Treatment and Care in China." Available at: http://www.unchina.org/unaids/.

Directorate General of Communicable Disease Control and Environmental Health. 2003. "National Estimates of HIV Among Adults in Indonesia, 2002: Report of a National Process to Estimate the Size of Populations at Risk for HIV." Jakarta.

Eberstadt, N. 2002. "The Future of AIDS." *Foreign Affairs* 81(6): 22–45.

Feng, C. Undated. "A Situation Assessment of Drug Use in China in the Context of HIV/AIDS." Chinese Center for Disease Prevention and Control, Beijing, and U.K. Department for International Development, London.

FHI/USAID (Family Health International/U.S. Agency for International Development). 2001a. "Effective Prevention Strategies in Low HIV Prevalence Settings." Arlington, Va.

———. 2001b. "Reducing Mother-to-Child Transmission: A Strategic Framework." Arlington, Va.

Garnett, G. 1998. "The Basic Reproductive Rate of Infection and the Course of HIV Epidemics." *AIDS Patient Care and STDs* 12(6): 435–449.

Global HIV Prevention Working Group. 2003. "Access to HIV Prevention: Closing the Gap." Geneva.

Gold, J., and E. Dax. 2003. "HIV Transmission by Blood Transfusion in Asia and the Pacific: Situation Analysis, National Responses and Policy—Programmatic Implications." World Bank, East Asia and Pacific Human Development Sector Unit, Washington, D.C.

Gold, J., and D. Smith. 2003. "Background Paper on Antiretroviral Therapy (ART Issues in East Asia and the Pacific Region)." World Bank, East Asia and Pacific Human Development Sector Unit, Washington, D.C.

Gold, J., and A. Wilson. 2002. "National Responses to HIV/AIDS in the East-Asia Pacific Region of the World Bank." World Bank, East Asia and Pacific Human Development Sector Unit, Washington, D.C.

Hickman, M., D. de Angelis, and S. Yang. 2003. "Progress in Estimating the Size of IDU Populations." Presented at the 14th International Conference on the Reduction of Drug Related Harm, April 6–10, Chiang Mai, Thailand.

Lin, V., and A. Heywood. 2002. "World Bank Lending and Sector Work for HIV/AIDS in East Asia and the Pacific: Review of Current and Past Activities and Strategies for the Future." World Bank, East Asia and Pacific Human Development Sector Unit, Washington, D.C.

NASB (National AIDS Standing Bureau). 2002. Internal report. Hanoi.

NASB/MOH. National AIDS Standing Bureau/Ministry of Health Report. 2003. Report. Hanoi.

Philippines Department of Health, Women's Health and Safe Motherhood Project, National AIDS/STD Prevention and Control Program, Philippine National AIDS Council Secretariat, Family Health International. 2002. "RTI/STI Prevalence in Selected Sites in the Philippines." Manila.

Pisani, E., S. Prihutomo, R. Pramoedyo, J. Djaelani, and Irwanto. 2003. "Progress in Estimating the Size of IDU Populations." Presented at the 14th International Conference on the Reduction of Drug Related Harm, April 6–10, Chiang Mai, Thailand.

Reid, G., and G. Costigan. 2002. "Revisiting the Hidden Epidemic." The Center for Harm Reduction, The Burnet Institute, Melbourne, Australia.

Rojanapithayakorn, W., and R. Hanenberg. 1996. "The 100% Condom Program in Thailand." *AIDS* 10(1): 1–7.

Schwarlander, B., K. Stanecki, T. Brown, P. Way, R. Monasch, J. Chin, D. Tarantola, and N. Walker. 1999. "Country-Specific Estimates and Models of HIV and AIDS: Methods and Limitations." *AIDS* 13: 2445–58.

Thai Working Group on HIV/AIDS Projections. 2001. *Projections for HIV/AIDS in Thailand: 2000–2020.* Thai Ministry of Public Health, Bangkok.

UNAIDS (Joint United Nations Programme on HIV/AIDS). 2000. *Report on the Global HIV/AIDS Epidemic.* Geneva.

———. 2002. *Report on the Global HIV/AIDS Epidemic.* Geneva.

UNAIDS/WHO (Joint United Nations Programme on HIV/AIDS/World Health Organization). 2000. "Second Generation Surveillance for HIV: The Next Decade." Geneva.

———. 2002. *Epidemiological Fact Sheets by Country: 2002 Updates.* Geneva.

UNAIDS/WHO/International HIV/AIDS Alliance. 2003. *Handbook on Access to HIV/AIDS Related Treatment.* Geneva.

USAID. Available at: http://www.usaid.gov/.

WHO (World Health Organization). 2001. *HIV/AIDS in Asia and the Pacific Region.* New Delhi and Manila.

———. 2003. *WHO Report 2003: Global Tuberculosis Control: Surveillance, Planning, Financing, World Health Organization.* Geneva.

World Bank. 1999. *Confronting AIDS: Public Priorities in a Global Epidemic.* Revised edition. New York: Oxford University Press.

———. 2000. *Thailand Social Monitor: Thailand's Response to AIDS: Building on Success, Confronting the Future.* Bangkok.

———. 2001. *World Development Indicators 2001.* Available at: worldbank.org (http://www.worldbank.org/data/wdi2001/).

———. 2002. *Education and HIV/AIDS: A Window of Hope.* Washington, D.C.

———. 2003. "HIV/AIDS in Indonesia: Strategy Note for New CAS." Washington, D.C.

Bibliography

Ainsworth, M., C. Beyrer, and A. Soucat. 2003. "AIDS and Public Policy: The Lessons and Challenges of 'Success' in Thailand." *Health Policy* 64: 13–37.

Anderson, R. 1996. "The Spread of HIV and Sexual Mixing Patterns." In J. Mann, ed., *AIDS in the World II. The Global Dimensions, Social Roots and Responses.* New York: Oxford University Press.

Anderson, R., R. May, M. Boily, G. Garnett, and J. Rowley. 1991. "The Spread of HIV-1 in Africa: Sexual Contact Patterns and the Predicted Demographic Impact of AIDS." *Nature* 352: 581–9.

Beeharry, G., N. Schwab, D. Akhavan, R. Hernandez, and C. Paredes. 2002. *Optimizing the Allocation of Resources Among HIV Prevention Interventions in Honduras.* HNP Discussion Paper. Washington, D.C.: World Bank.

Brown, T. 2002. "HIV/AIDS in Asia: The Future of Population in Asia." East-West Center, Honolulu.

Brown, T., and P. Xenos. 1994. "AIDS in Asia: The Gathering Storm." *AsiaPacific Issues* 16: 1–15.

Chin, J. 1990. "Public Health Surveillance of AIDS and HIV Infections." *Bulletin of the World Health Organization* 68(5): 529–36.

———. 1995. "Scenarios for the AIDS Epidemic in Asia." *East-West Center Asia-Pacific Population Research Reports, No. 2.* Honolulu: East-West Center.

———. 2001. "The Past, Present and Probable Future of AIDS in Asia." Presented at the U.K. Department for International Development Asia Health Retreat, May 20–22, Bangkok.

———. 2002. "Assessing the HIV/AIDS Pandemic Using a New Paradigm: The Collision of Epidemiology with Political Correctness." Presented at the annual meeting of the American Epidemiological Society, March 20–23, New York.

Chin, J., A. Bennett, and S. Mills. 1998. "Primary Determinants of HIV Prevalence in Asian-Pacific Countries." *AIDS* 12(Suppl. B): S87–S91.

CSR/WHO (Communicable Disease Surveillance and Response/World Health Organization). 2003. "SARS: Status of the Outbreak and Lessons for the Immediate Future." Geneva.

Dhingra, N. 2003. "SARS as an Emerging Pathogen." World Health Organization Global Conference on SARS, June 17–18, Kuala Lumpur.

Dore, G., T. Brown, D. Tarantola, and J. Kaldor. 1998. "HIV and AIDS in the Asia-Pacific Region: An Epidemiological Overview." *AIDS* 12(Suppl. B): S1–S10.

Garcia-Abreu, A., I. Noguer, and K. Cowgill. 2002. "HIV/AIDS in Latin America: The Challenges Ahead." World Bank, Human Development Network, Washington, D.C.

Haque, S. 2002. "Non-financial Constraints in Scaling up HIV/AIDS Interventions: Case Studies of Cambodia and China." World Bank, East Asia and Pacific Human Development Sector Unit, Washington, D.C.

Human Rights Watch. 2003. "Locked Doors: The Human Rights of People Living with HIV/AIDS in China." *HRW Report*, August, 15(7).

Khorloo, E. 2003. "Overview of HIV/AIDS and Drug Use in Mongolia." Presented at the China Plus Meeting I, April 6–10, Chiang Mai, Thailand.

National Intelligence Council. 2002. "The Next Wave of HIV/AIDS: Nigeria, Ethiopia, Russia, India and China." Washington, D.C.

Pisani, E., G. Garnett, T. Brown, J. Stover, N. Grassly, C. Hankins, N. Walker, and P. Ghys. 2003. "Back to Basics in HIV Prevention: Focus on Exposure." *BMJ* 326: 1384–7.

UNAIDS Interagency Task Team on Education. 2002. *HIV and Education: A Strategic Approach.* Paris.

WHO (World Health Organization). 2002. "Improving Health Outcomes of the Poor." Report of Working Group 5 of the Commission on Macroeconomics and Health. Geneva.

World Bank. 1997. *Health, Nutrition & Population.* Washington, D.C.

———. 1998. *Confronting AIDS: Evidence from the Developing World.* Brussels: European Commission.

———. 2000. *Statistical Information Management and Analysis: GDF and WDI Central Databases.* Washington, D.C.

———. 2002a. *Public Health and World Bank Operations.* Washington, D.C.

———. 2002b. *Public Health Surveillance Toolkit.* Washington, D.C.

———. 2002c. *The Multi-Country HIV/AIDS Program for Africa (MAP): Intensifying Action Against HIV/AIDS in Africa.* (CD-ROM). Washington, D.C.

———. 2003. *Averting AIDS Crises in Eastern Europe and Central Asia: A Regional Support Strategy.* Europe and Central Asia Region. Washington, D.C.

Web Sites

Asian Development Bank, http://www.adb.org/
AusAID, http://www.ausaid.gov.au/
Development Gateway, http://www.developmentgateway.org/
DFID, http://www.dfid.gov.uk/
Global Fund to Fight AIDS, Tuberculosis and Malaria,
    http://www.globalfundatm.org/
JICA, http://www.jica.go.jp/
KFW, http://www.kfw.de/DE/
UNAIDS, http://www.unaids.org/
UNDP, http://www.undp.org/
UNICEF, http://www.unicef.org/
USAID, http://www.usaid.gov/
World Bank, http://www.worldbank.org/
World Bank, *World Development Indicators,*
    http://www.worldbank.org/data/wdi2001/
World Health Organization, http://www.who.int/en/

Index

Page references followed by *t*, *f*, and *n* refer to tables, figures, and notes respectively.

A

ADB. *See* Asian Development Bank
AEM. *See* Asian Epidemic Model
Analytic and advisory work
  increasing need for, 6, 7, 39, 40, 42
  in World Bank anti-HIV/AIDS
    strategy, 9, 45
  World Bank role in, 6, 9, 39, 40,
    45, 46–47
Antiretrovirals
  defined, *xiii*
  demand for, 7, 9, 34
  maximizing effectiveness of, 8–9, 34
  number of patients receiving
    in Cambodia, 34, 53
    in China, 56
    in Indonesia, 57
    in Lao PDR, 61
    in Malaysia, 58
    in Mongolia, 62
    in Myanmar, 54
    in Papua New Guinea, 59
    in Philippines, 63
    in Thailand, 22, 34, 55
    in Vietnam, 60

  in prevention of mother-child
    transmission, 35
ASEAN. *See* Association of Southeast
  Asian Nations
Asian Development Bank (ADB)
  anti-HIV/AIDS programs, 5, 23,
    41, 53
  Web site, 97
Asian economic crisis, impact of, 3, 4,
  22, 24
Asian Epidemic Model (AEM)
  development of, 15–16, 76–77
  predictions for Cambodia, 16
  predictions for Thailand, 16, 21,
    77, 88*n*
Association of Southeast Asian Na-
  tions (ASEAN)
  anti-HIV/AIDS programs, 41
  Seventh Summit, 19
Australian anti-HIV/AIDS programs
  AusAID, 40, 54, 55, 56, 57, 59, 60,
    61, 62
  Web site, 97
  domestic, 32–33

B

Blood supply
  HIV/AIDS transmission by
    in China, 56

Blood supply (*cont.*)
   HIV/AIDS transmission by (*cont.*)
     in Indonesia, 57
     in Malaysia, 58
     in Myanmar, 54
     in Papua New Guinea, 59
     in Philippines, 63
   safety of
     in Cambodia, 53, 81*t*
     in China, 5, 27, 38, 56, 82*t*
     in Indonesia, 57, 82*t*
     in Lao PDR, 61, 83*t*
     in Malaysia, 58, 82*t*
     in Mongolia, 62, 83*t*
     monitoring, 31, 45
     in Papua New Guinea, 59, 82*t*–83*t*
     in Philippines, 63, 84*t*
     in Vietnam, 60
Brown, Tim, 15–16, 76
Bureaucracy for HIV/AIDS policy
   importance of, 5, 6, 7, 26, 29–30,
     41–42
   Indonesia, 4, 24, 29–30
   Papua New Guinea, 4, 26
   Thailand, 20–21, 29

C
Cambodia
   antiretroviral patients, 34, 53
   blood supply safety in, 53, 81*t*
   drug use, intravenous, 66*t*
   Global Fund funding, 53, 85*t*
   GNI per capita, 12*t*, 53
   mode of HIV transmission, 53
   multidrug resistance in, 53
   national health accounts in, 43
   NGOs in, 34
   number of HIV/AIDS-infected
     persons, 12*t*, 18*t*
   population, 12*t*, 18*t*, 53
   prevalence of HIV/AIDS, 11–14,
     12*t*, 18*t*, 23, 50*f*, 53, 66*t*
     predicted trends in, 16
   response to HIV/AIDS, 23, 32
     funding of, 53, 85*t*

   sex workers
     HIV/AIDS prevalence, 12*t*, 53, 68*t*
     number and characteristics of, 68*t*
   treatment programs in, 34
   tuberculosis in
     incidence, 53, 79*f*
     number of infected persons, 18*t*
     percent of infected persons also
      with HIV/AIDS, 53
     treatment of, 42–43
   World Bank anti-HIV/AIDS pro-
     grams, 53
Canada, anti-HIV/AIDS programs,
   32–33
CDC. *See* U.S. Centers for Disease
   Control and Prevention
Children and youth
   impact of HIV/AIDS on, 3, 17, 35,
     43
   incidence of HIV/AIDS, 33
   orphaned, care of, 35
China
   antiretroviral patients, 56
   blood supply safety in, 5, 27, 38,
     56, 82*t*
   drug treatment programs, 33
   drug use, intravenous, 56, 66*t*
   Global Fund funding, 56, 85*t*
   GNI per capita, 12*t*, 56
   incidence of HIV/AIDS, predicted
     trends in, 1, 5, 16, 27, 33, 75, 76
   mode of HIV transmission, 56
   multidrug resistance in, 56
   number of HIV/AIDS-infected
     persons, 11, 12*t*, 18*t*
   population, 12*t*, 18*t*, 56
   prevalence of HIV/AIDS, 12*t*, 14,
     18*t*, 50*f*, 56, 66*t*
   prevalence of SDIs, 76
   response to HIV/AIDS, 5, 27, 40,
     56
     funding of, 37–38, 56, 85*t*
   sex workers
     HIV/AIDS prevalence, 12*t*, 56, 68*t*
     number and characteristics of, 68*t*
   surveillance in, 30–31, 41

tuberculosis in
  incidence, 56, 79*f*
  number of infected persons, 18*t*
  percent of infected persons also
    with HIV/AIDS, 56
  treatment measures, 18
  World Bank anti-HIV/AIDS
    efforts in, 56
CIA. *See* U.S. Central Intelligence
  Agency
Commercial sex workers (CSWs). *See*
  Sex workers
Condom use
  programs to encourage, 20, 23, 32
  rate of
    Cambodia, 23
    Thailand, 21, 21*f*
Control of HIV/AIDS epidemic,
  complicating factors, *vii*
CSWs (commercial sex workers). *See*
  Sex workers

D

Data on HIV/AIDS, limitations of, 2,
  6, 8, 11, 31, 44, 51
Death, leading cause of, in
  HIV/AIDS, 2
Department for International Devel-
  opment (DFID)
  anti-HIV/AIDS programs, 18, 23,
    40, 53, 54, 56, 60
  Web site, 97
Development Gateway, Web site, 97
DFID. *See* Department for Interna-
  tional Development
Directly Observed Therapy, Short-
  Course (DOTS), 18
Discrimination against HIV/AIDS-
  infected persons, legal reforms to
  reduce, 3–4, 23, 30, 34
DOTS. *See* Directly Observed Ther-
  apy, Short-Course
Drug treatment programs, 33
  in China, 56
  in Indonesia, 57
  in Myanmar, 54

  in Philippines, 63
  in Thailand, 55
Drug users, intravenous
  access to prevention programs, 32
  HIV/AIDS prevention programs
    for, 4, 22, 25, 30, 32–33, 43–44
  HIV/AIDS transmission by
    in China, 56
    in Indonesia, 57
    in Malaysia, 58
    in Myanmar, 54
    in Philippines, 63
    in Thailand, 55
    in Vietnam, 60
  number and characteristics of, 14, 44
    in Cambodia, 66*t*
    in China, 56, 66*t*
    in Indonesia, 57, 66*t*
    in Lao PDR, 67*t*
    in Malaysia, 67*t*
    in Mongolia, 67*t*
    in Myanmar, 54, 66*t*
    in Philippines, 63, 67*t*
    in Thailand, 55, 66*t*
    in Vietnam, 60, 67*t*
  as origin of HIV/AIDS, 2, 14, 87*n*
  prevalence of HIV/AIDS, 14
    in Cambodia, 12*t*, 14, 53, 66*t*
    in China, 12*t*, 56, 66*t*
    in Indonesia, 4, 12*t*, 25, 57, 66*t*
    in Lao PDR, 13*t*, 61, 67*t*
    in Malaysia, 12*t*, 58, 67*t*
    in Mongolia, 13*t*, 62, 67*t*
    in Myanmar, 12*t*, 54, 66*t*
    in Papua New Guinea, 12*t*, 59
    in Philippines, 13*t*, 24, 63, 67*t*
    in Thailand, 3, 12*t*, 22, 55, 66*t*
    in Vietnam, 12*t*, 60, 67*t*

E

Eberstadt, Nicholas, 75, 76*t*, 89*n*–90*n*
Economic development, impact of
  HIV/AIDS on, 3, 17, 43, 75
Ensemble pur une Solidarité
  Thérapeutique Hospitalière en
  Réseau, 34

Epidemic. *See also* Models of
HIV/AIDS spread; Spread of
HIV/AIDS
defined, *xiii*
generalized, defined, 2
of HIV/AIDS
magnitude, by nation, 2, 11–14,
12*t*–13*t*, 50*f*
risk level, by nation, *xvif*
of tuberculosis, potential for, 2
Epidemiology of HIV/AIDS. *See also*
Models of HIV/AIDS spread;
Spread of HIV/AIDS
in Indonesia, 4, 25
in Thailand, 21–22

F
French Cooperation, anti-HIV/AIDS
programs, 53

G
Germany, anti-HIV/AIDS programs,
32–33
GFATM. *See* Global Fund to Fight
AIDS, Tuberculosis, and Malaria
Global Fund to Fight AIDS, Tuberculosis, and Malaria (GFATM)
projects funded by, 5, 6, 36, 40,
85*t*–86*t*
in Cambodia, 53, 85*t*
in China, 56, 85*t*
in Indonesia, 57, 86*t*
in Lao PDR, 61, 86*t*
in Mongolia, 62, 86*t*
in Myanmar, 54, 85*t*
in Philippines, 63, 86*t*
in Thailand, 55, 85*t*
in Vietnam, 60, 86*t*
Web site, 97
Global HIV/AIDS Monitoring and
Evaluation Support Team, 8
Global program on AIDS, anti-
HIV/AIDS programs, 26
GNI. *See* Gross national income
(GNI) per capita

Gross national income (GNI) per
capita, 12*t*–13*t*
Cambodia, 12*t*, 53
China, 12*t*, 56
Indonesia, 12*t*, 57
Lao PDR, 13*t*, 61
Malaysia, 12*t*, 58
Mongolia, 13*t*, 62
Myanmar, 12*t*, 54
Papua New Guinea, 12*t*, 59
Philippines, 13*t*, 63
Thailand, 12*t*, 55
Vietnam, 12*t*, 60

H
Harm reduction policies, 32–33, 40
Health care systems. *See also* Treatment of HIV/AIDS
impact of Asian economic crisis on,
3, 4, 22, 24
impact of HIV/AIDS on, 2–3, 17,
25, 35–36, 43
in Indonesia, 24
in Thailand, 22
impact of SARS on, 25
improvement of, 7, 35–36, 44–45
funding for, 37–38
in World Bank anti-HIV/AIDS
strategy, 9, 44–45
Homosexuals
HIV/AIDS prevention programs
for, 22, 30, 33
number of, as key to future of epidemic, 14
as origin of HIV/AIDS, 2
prevalence of HIV/AIDS in, 24
transmission of HIV/AIDS by
in China, 56
in Indonesia, 57
in Malaysia, 58
in Mongolia, 62
in Myanmar, 54
in Papua New Guinea, 59
in Philippines, 63
in Thailand, 55

Hong Kong, drug treatment program, 33
Human rights. *See* Discrimination against HIV/AIDS-infected persons

I

IBRD. *See* International Bank for Reconstruction and Development
IDA. *See* International Development Association
Incidence of HIV/AIDS
  in children and youth, 33
  as key to future of epidemic, 14
  predicted trends in, 1–3, 15–16, 75–77. *See also* Models of HIV/AIDS spread
  and anti-HIV/AIDS program design, 8, 42–43
  China, 1, 5, 16, 27, 33, 75, 76
  Indonesia, 1, 16, 33, 76
  Malaysia, 76
  Papua New Guinea, 16, 76
  Russia, 75
  Thailand, 16, 21, 33, 77, 88*n*
  Vietnam, 76
Incidence rate, defined, *xiii*
India, prevalence of HIV/AIDS in, 1, 75
Indonesia
  antiretroviral patients, 57
  blood supply safety in, 57, 82*t*
  drug treatment programs, 33
  drug use, intravenous, 57, 66*t*
  Global Fund funding, 57, 86*t*
  GNI per capita, 12*t*, 57
  incidence of HIV/AIDS, predicted trends in, 1, 16, 33, 76
  mode of HIV transmission, 57
  multidrug resistance in, 57
  national health accounts in, 43
  number of HIV/AIDS-infected persons, 12*t*, 18*t*
  population, 12*t*, 18*t*, 57
  prevalence of HIV/AIDS, 4, 12*t*, 14, 18*t*, 24, 25, 50*f*, 57, 66*t*

prevalence of SDIs, 76
response to HIV/AIDS, 4, 24–25, 29–30, 38, 40
  funding of, 37, 57, 86*t*
sex workers
  HIV/AIDS prevalence, 12, 25, 57, 68*t*
  number and characteristics of, 68*t*
surveillance in, 24, 31
tuberculosis in
  incidence, 57, 79*f*
  number of infected persons, 18*t*
  percent of infected persons also with HIV/AIDS, 57
World Bank anti-HIV/AIDS efforts in, 57
Influenza, epidemiology, 71
International Bank for Reconstruction and Development (IBRD), 45
International Development Association (IDA), 45

J

Japan International Cooperation Agency (JICA)
  anti-HIV/AIDS programs, 40, 53, 54, 55, 58, 61, 63
  web site, 97
Joint United Nationals Program on HIV/AIDS (UNAIDS)
  on access to anti-HIV/AIDS programs, 32
  on AIDS orphans, 17
  anti-HIV/AIDS programs, 5, 23, 40, 41, 53
  best practice dissemination, 46–47
  on cost of preventing spread of HIV/AIDS, 38
  HIV/AIDS data, 2, 11, 51
  models of HIV/AIDS epidemiology, 77
  predicted spread of HIV/AIDS, 1–2, 16, 17*f*
  Web site, 97

K

KFW Bankengruppe
   anti-HIV/AIDS programs, 57
   Web site, 97

L

Lao PDR
   antiretroviral patients, 61
   blood supply safety in, 61, 83t
   drug use, intravenous, 67t
   Global Fund funding, 61, 86t
   GNI per capita, 13t, 61
   mode of HIV transmission, 61
   number of HIV/AIDS-infected
      persons, 13t, 18t
   population, 13t, 18t, 61
   prevalence of HIV/AIDS, 13t, 14,
      18t, 50f, 61, 67t
   response to HIV/AIDS, 61
      funding of, 61, 86t
   sex workers
      HIV/AIDS prevalence, 13t, 61, 69t
      number and characteristics of, 69t
   tuberculosis in
      incidence, 61, 79f
      number of infected persons, 18t
Leaders and public figures, anti-
   HIV/AIDS programs and, 30
London School of Hygiene and
   Tropical Medicine, on cost of
   prevention, 38

M

Malaysia
   antiretroviral patients, 58
   blood supply safety in, 58, 82t
   drug use, intravenous, 67t
   GNI per capita, 12t, 58
   incidence of HIV/AIDS, predicted
      trends in, 76
   mode of HIV transmission, 58
   number of HIV/AIDS-infected
      persons, 12t, 18t
   population, 12t, 18t, 58
   prevalence of HIV/AIDS, 12t, 14,
      18t, 50f, 58, 67t

prevalence of SDIs, 76
sex workers
   HIV/AIDS prevalence, 12t, 58, 69t
   number and characteristics of, 69t
tuberculosis in
   incidence, 58, 79f
   number of infected persons, 18t
World Bank anti-HIV/AIDS
   efforts in, 58
Men
   percent of sex worker use, 14, 21,
      73, 76, 77
   practicing homosexuals
      HIV/AIDS prevention programs
         for, 22, 30, 33
      number of, as key to future of
         epidemic, 14
      as origin of HIV/AIDS, 2
      prevalence of HIV/AIDS, 24
      transmission of HIV/AIDS by
         in China, 56
         in Indonesia, 57
         in Malaysia, 58
         in Mongolia, 62
         in Myanmar, 54
         in Papua New Guinea, 59
         in Philippines, 63
         in Thailand, 55
      rate of sex outside of long-term
         relationships, 16, 21, 77
      with STDs, HIV prevalence, by
         nation, 12t–13t
Migration, and spread of HIV/AIDS,
   14–15, 33, 41
Models of HIV/AIDS spread, 71–73,
   72f, 89n
   Asian Epidemic Model
      development of, 15–16, 76–77
      predictions for Cambodia, 16
      predictions for Thailand, 16, 21,
         77, 88n
   Eberstadt model, 75, 76t, 89n–90n
   UNAIDS model, 77
Mongolia
   antiretroviral patients, 62
   blood supply safety in, 62, 83t

drug use, intravenous, 67*t*
Global Fund funding, 62, 86*t*
GNI per capita, 13*t*, 62
mode of HIV transmission, 62
number of HIV/AIDS-infected
    persons, 13*t*, 18*t*
population, 13*t*, 18*t*, 62
prevalence of HIV/AIDS, 13*t*, 14,
    18*t*, 50*f*, 62, 67*t*
response to HIV/AIDS, funding of,
    62, 86*t*
sex workers
    HIV/AIDS prevalence, 13*t*, 62,
        69*t*
    number and characteristics of,
        62, 69*t*
tuberculosis in
    incidence, 62, 79*f*
    number of infected persons, 18*t*
Monitoring
    of anti-HIV/AIDS programs, 32,
        38–39
    of spread of HIV/AIDS. *See also*
        Surveillance
    approaches to, 6, 31
    for recurrence, 22
    in World Bank anti-HIV/AIDS
        strategy, 8, 43
Myanmar
    antiretroviral patients, 54
    drug use, intravenous, 54, 66*t*
    Global Fund funding, 54, 85*t*
    GNI per capita, 12*t*, 54
    mode of HIV transmission, 54
    multidrug resistance in, 54
    number of HIV/AIDS-infected
        persons, 12*t*, 14, 18*t*
    population, 12*t*, 18*t*, 54
    prevalence of HIV/AIDS, 11–14,
        12*t*, 18*t*, 50*f*, 54, 66*t*
    response to HIV/AIDS, 40
        funding of, 54, 85*t*
    sex workers
        HIV/AIDS prevalence, 12*t*, 54,
            68*t*
        number and characteristics of, 68*t*

tuberculosis in
    incidence, 54, 79*f*
    number of infected persons, 18*t*
    percent of infected persons also
        with HIV/AIDS, 54

N
National Center for HIV/AIDS,
    Dermatology, and STD
    (NCHADS), 42–43, 53
National health accounts, 8, 43
NCHADS. *See* National Center for
    HIV/AIDS, Dermatology, and
    STD
Netherlands, anti-HIV/AIDS pro-
    grams, 32–33
NGOs. *See* Nongovernmental
    organizations
Nongovernmental organizations
    (NGOs)
    anti-HIV/AIDS programs, 5, 30
    efficacy of, 39
    in Indonesia, 4, 24
    in Thailand, 20
    implementation support for, 39
    treatment programs
        in Cambodia, 34
        in World Bank anti-HIV/AIDS
            strategy, 44
Number of HIV/AIDS-infected
    persons
    Cambodia, 12*t*, 18*t*
    China, 11, 12*t*, 18*t*
    in EAP Region, 11
    Indonesia, 12*t*, 18*t*
    Lao PDR, 13*t*, 18*t*
    Malaysia, 12*t*, 18*t*
    Mongolia, 13*t*, 18*t*
    Myanmar, 12*t*, 14, 18*t*
    Papua New Guinea, 12*t*, 18*t*
    Philippines, 13*t*, 18*t*
        percent returning from abroad, 15
    Thailand, 12*t*, 18*t*
    Tuvalu, 11
    Vietnam, 12*t*, 18*t*
    worldwide, 11

O

OECD. *See* Organisation for Economic Co-operation and Development
Opportunistic infections
defined, *xiii*
increased risk in HIV/AIDS, 2, 16–17
Chinese health measures and, 18
treatment of, 22, 35
Organisation for Economic Co-operation and Development (OECD), 36

P

Pacific Island Member States
members, 87*n*
prevalence of HIV/AIDS, 14
Pandemic, defined, *xiii*
Papua New Guinea
antiretroviral patients, 59
blood supply safety in, 59
GNI per capita, 12*t*, 59
incidence of HIV/AIDS, predicted trends in, 16, 76
mode of HIV transmission, 59
number of HIV/AIDS-infected persons, 12*t*, 18*t*
population, 12*t*, 18*t*, 59
prevalence of HIV/AIDS, 11, 12*t*, 14, 18*t*, 50*f*, 59
response to HIV/AIDS, 4, 25–26, 59
risk factors for epidemic in, 4, 25–26
sex workers
HIV/AIDS prevalence, 12*t*, 59, 69*t*
number and characteristics of, 69*t*
spread of HIV/AIDS in, 26
surveillance in, 4, 26
tuberculosis in
incidence, 59, 79*f*
number of infected persons, 18*t*
World Bank anti-HIV/AIDS efforts in, 59
Papua New Guinea, blood supply safety in, 82*t*–83*t*
Peerapatinapokin, Wiwat, 15–16, 76

Philippines
antiretroviral patients, 63
blood supply safety in, 63, 84*t*
drug use, intravenous, 63, 67*t*
Global Fund funding, 63, 86*t*
GNI per capita, 13*t*, 63
mode of HIV transmission, 63
multidrug resistance in, 63
number of HIV/AIDS-infected persons, 13*t*, 18*t*
percent returned from abroad, 15
population, 13*t*, 18*t*, 63
prevalence of HIV/AIDS, 13*t*, 14, 18*t*, 24, 50*f*, 63, 67*t*
response to HIV/AIDS, 3–4, 23–24, 63
funding of, 63, 86*t*
sex workers
HIV/AIDS prevalence, 13*t*, 24, 63, 69*t*
number and characteristics of, 69*t*
surveillance in, 23, 24
tuberculosis in
incidence, 63, 79*f*
number of infected persons, 18*t*
percent of infected persons also with HIV/AIDS, 63
Population, 12*t*, 18*t*
Cambodia, 12*t*, 18*t*, 53
China, 12*t*, 18*t*, 56
of EAP Region, 11
Indonesia, 12*t*, 18*t*, 57
Lao PDR, 13*t*, 18*t*, 61
Malaysia, 12*t*, 18*t*, 58
Mongolia, 13*t*, 18*t*, 62
Myanmar, 12*t*, 18*t*, 54
Papua New Guinea, 12*t*, 18*t*, 59
Philippines, 13*t*, 18*t*, 63
Thailand, 12*t*, 18*t*, 55
Timor Leste, 18*t*
Vietnam, 12*t*, 18*t*, 60
Prevalence of HIV/AIDS, 11–14, 12*t*–13*t*, 15*f*
Cambodia, 11–14, 12*t*, 18*t*, 23, 50*f*, 53, 63*t*
predicted trends in, 16
China, 12*t*, 14, 18*t*, 50*f*, 56, 66*t*

India, 1, 75
Indonesia, 4, 12*t*, 14, 18*t*, 24, 25,
    50*f*, 57, 66*t*
Lao PDR, 13*t*, 14, 18*t*, 50*f*, 61, 67*t*
Malaysia, 12*t*, 14, 18*t*, 50*f*, 58, 67*t*
Mongolia, 13*t*, 14, 18*t*, 50*f*, 62, 67*t*
Myanmar, 11–14, 12*t*, 18*t*, 50*f*, 54,
    66*t*
Pacific Island Member States, 14
Papua New Guinea, 11, 12*t*, 14,
    18*t*, 50*f*, 59
Philippines, 13*t*, 14, 18*t*, 24, 50*f*,
    63, 67*t*
Thailand, 3, 11–14, 12*t*, 18*t*,
    19–20, 21, 50*f*, 55, 66*t*
Timor Leste, 14
Vietnam, 12*t*, 14, 18*t*, 50*f*, 60, 67*t*
Prevalence rate, defined, *xiii*, 88*n*
Prevention of HIV/AIDS. *See also*
    Prevention programs
  cost of, 38
    projecting, 73
  current spending on, 38
Prevention programs
  access to, 32
  approaches to, 6, 32–34
  Cambodia, 23, 32
  China, 5, 27, 40, 56
    funding of, 37–38, 56, 85*t*
  funding of, 3, 4, 5–6, 22, 23, 24, 26,
    30, 37–38, 39–41, 85*t*–86*t*
  groups requiring special attention, 33
  harm reduction programs, 32–33, 40
  implementation *vs.* design of, 38–39
  importance of maintaining, 8, 22, 24
  Indonesia, 4, 24–25, 29–30, 37, 40
  Lao PDR, 61
  lessons learned in, 4–5, 26–27, 39
  monitoring of, 8, 31–32, 38–39, 43
  multisector involvement in, 7, 36,
    38, 41–42
  Myanmar, 40
  Papua New Guinea, 4, 25–26, 59
  Philippines, 3–4, 23–24, 63
  political support for
    importance of, 5, 6, 7, 26, 29–30,
      41–42

  in Indonesia, 4, 24, 29
  in Papua New Guinea, 4, 26
  in Thailand, 20–21, 29
  Thailand, 3, 19–21, 29, 32, 33, 39, 41
    success of, 3, 21–22, 21*f*
  Vietnam, 27, 37, 40
  in World Bank anti-HIV/AIDS
    strategy, 8, 43–44
Prisoners, prevention strategies for, 33
Public information campaigns
  importance of, 7, 29, 33, 42
  in Thailand, 20
Public opinion, importance of
    gauging, 42

R
Reporting requirements for
    HIV/AIDS case, in Thailand, 20
Reproductive rate, 71–73, 72*f*
  defined, *xiii*
Resistance, multidrug
  in Cambodia, 53
  in China, 56
  in Indonesia, 57
  in Myanmar, 54
  in Philippines, 63
  in Thailand, 55
  in Vietnam, 60
Response to HIV/AIDS. *See also* Pre-
    vention programs; Treatment of
    HIV/AIDS
  public commitments to, 5, 19, 27
Risk behaviors. *See also* Drug users,
    intravenous; Sex workers
  and access to anti-HIV/AIDS pro-
    grams, 32
  efforts to decrease, 20–21, 30, 38, 40
  in general population, 15
  risk of HIV infection and, 22
  size of population practicing, 2, 14,
    16, 75–76, 77
    importance of ascertaining, 6,
      7–8, 31, 42
  as key to future trends, 14
  spread to general population from,
    1–2, 3, 5, 15–16, 19–20, 27,
    71, 77*f*

Russia, incidence of HIV/AIDS, predicted trends in, 75

S
SARS. *See* Severe acute respiratory syndrome
Severe acute respiratory syndrome (SARS)
  epidemiology, 71
  impact on health care systems, 25
Sex workers
  HIV/AIDS prevention programs for, 3, 20–21, 22, 23, 24, 25, 30, 32, 43–44
  number and characteristics of, 14, 44
    in Cambodia, 68*t*
    in China, 68*t*
    in Indonesia, 68*t*
    in Lao PDR, 69*t*
    in Malaysia, 69*t*
    in Mongolia, 69*t*
    in Myanmar, 68*t*
    in Papua New Guinea, 69*t*
    in Philippines, 69*t*
    in Thailand, 68*t*
    in Vietnam, 69*t*
  as origin of HIV/AIDS, 2, 14, 87*n*
  percent of males using, 14, 21, 73, 76, 77
  prevalence of HIV/AIDS, 14
    in Cambodia, 12*t*, 53, 68*t*
    in China, 12*t*, 56, 68*t*
    in Indonesia, 12*t*, 25, 57, 68*t*
    in Lao PDR, 13*t*, 61, 69*t*
    in Malaysia, 12*t*, 58, 69*t*
    in Mongolia, 13*t*, 62, 69*t*
    in Myanmar, 12*t*, 54, 68*t*
    in Papua New Guinea, 12*t*, 59, 69*t*
    in Philippines, 13*t*, 24, 63, 69*t*
    in Thailand, 3, 12*t*, 19–20, 55, 68*t*
    in Vietnam, 12*t*, 60, 69*t*
Sexually transmitted diseases (STDs)
  checking sex workers for, 20–21
  control of, 33
  incidence
    in Philippines, 3, 24
    Thailand, 21, 21*f*, 33

males with, HIV prevalence
    in Cambodia, 12*t*, 53
    in China, 12*t*, 56
    in Indonesia, 12*t*, 57
    in Lao PDR, 13*t*, 61
    in Malaysia, 12*t*, 58
    in Mongolia, 13*t*, 62
    in Myanmar, 12*t*, 54
    in Papua New Guinea, 12*t*, 59
    in Philippines, 13*t*, 63
    in Thailand, 12*t*, 55
    in Vietnam, 12*t*, 60
  prevalence
    in China, 76
    in Indonesia, 76
    in Malaysia, 76
    in Vietnam, 76
  as proxy for HIV/AIDS, 31
Social fabric, impact of HIV/AIDS on, 3, 17
Spread of HIV/AIDS. *See also* Models of HIV/AIDS spread
  factors affecting, 14–15, 33, 41, 71–73, 72*f*
  from high-risk population to general population, 1–2, 3, 5, 15–16, 19–20, 27
  monitoring of. *See also* Surveillance
    approaches to, 6, 8, 30–31
    for recurrence, 22
    in Papua New Guinea, 26
  predictions for, 1–3, 15–16, 75–77
    and anti-HIV/AIDS program design, 8, 42–43
    by UNAIDS, 16
  prevention of. *See* Prevention
STDs. *See* Sexually transmitted diseases
Surveillance
  behavioral, 3, 20, 23, 24, 31, 42
  defined, *xiii*
  in China, 31, 41
  development of, 4, 24, 26, 38, 41, 46
  funding of, 31, 38
  of general population, 31
  of high risk behaviors, 31

importance of maintaining, 22, 24, 26
in Indonesia, 24, 31
as key to effective programs, 6,
   31–32
in Papua New Guinea, 4, 26
in Philippines, 23, 24
sentinel HIV, 3, 4, 20, 23, 31, 42
   defined, *xiv*
serological, 3, 20
in Thailand, 3, 20, 22
in United States, 41
in Vietnam, 31, 41
in World Bank strategy, 7–8, 42–43
Switzerland, anti-HIV/AIDS programs, 32–33

T

Thailand
antiretroviral patients, 22, 34, 55
drug use, intravenous, 55, 66*t*
Global Fund funding, 55, 85*t*
GNI per capita, 12*t*, 55
health care systems, impact of
   HIV/AIDS on, 17, 22
high-risk behavior in, 77
incidence of HIV/AIDS, predicted
   trends in, 16, 21, 33, 77, 88*n*
incidence of STDs, 21, 21*f*, 33
mode of HIV transmission, 55
multidrug resistance in, 55
number of HIV/AIDS-infected
   persons, 12*t*, 18*t*
population, 12*t*, 18*t*, 55
prevalence of HIV/AIDS, 3, 11–14,
   12*t*, 18*t*, 19–20, 21, 50*f*, 55, 66*t*
response to HIV/AIDS, 3, 19–21,
   30, 32, 33, 39, 41
   efficacy of, 3, 21–22, 21*f*
   funding of, 55, 85*t*
sex workers
   HIV/AIDS prevalence, 3, 12*t*,
      19–20, 55, 68*t*
   number and characteristics of, 68*t*
spending on HIV/AIDS preven-
   tion, 38
surveillance in, 3, 20, 22

treatment programs in, 34
tuberculosis in
   incidence, 55, 79*f*
   number of infected persons, 18*t*
   percent of infected persons also
      with HIV/AIDS, 55
World Bank anti-HIV/AIDS efforts in, 55
Thailand Social Monitor: Thailand's Re-
   sponse to AIDS: Building on Suc-
   cess, Confronting the Future
   (World Bank), 39
Timor Leste
   number of HIV/AIDS-infected
      persons, 18*t*
   population, 18*t*
   prevalence of HIV/AIDS, 14, 18*t*
   tuberculosis, number of infected
      persons, 18*t*
Transmission of HIV/AIDS
   likelihood of, 72–73
   mode of
      in Cambodia, 53
      in China, 56
      in Indonesia, 57
      in Lao PDR, 61
      in Malaysia, 58
      in Mongolia, 62
      in Myanmar, 54
      in Papua New Guinea, 59
      in Philippines, 63
      in Thailand, 55
      in Vietnam, 60
Treatment of HIV/AIDS. *See also*
   Antiretrovirals; Health care systems; Opportunistic infections
   access to, 36, 40
   adequacy of, 36
   counseling and referral, 4, 7, 23,
      34, 35
   funding of, 36
   goals of, 34
   importance of, 30
   NGOs and, 34, 44
   planning for, 8–9, 42–43
   private spending on, 38, 44

Treatment of HIV/AIDS (*cont.*)
  programs and methods, 7, 22,
    34–35, 44
  reporting systems for, 32
  in World Bank anti-HIV/AIDS
    strategy, 8–9, 44
Treatment of tuberculosis
  methods, 18, 35
  planning for, 42–43
Tuberculosis
  in Cambodia
    incidence, 53, 79*f*
    number of infected persons, 18*t*
    percent of infected persons also
      with HIV/AIDS, 53
    treatment of, 42–43
  in China
    incidence, 56, 79*f*
    number of infected persons, 18*t*
    percent of infected persons also
      with HIV/AIDS, 56
    preventive measures, 18
  in EAP Region, 16–17
  increased risk in HIV/AIDS, 2, 16–17
  in Indonesia
    incidence, 57, 79*f*
    number of infected persons, 18*t*
    percent of infected persons also
      with HIV/AIDS, 57
  in Lao PDR
    incidence, 61, 79*f*
    number of infected persons, 18*t*
  as leading cause of death in
    HIV/AIDS, 2
  in Malaysia
    incidence, 58, 79*f*
    number of infected persons, 18*t*
  in Mongolia
    incidence, 62, 79*f*
    number of infected persons, 18*t*
  in Myanmar
    incidence, 54, 79*f*
    number of infected persons, 18*t*
    percent of infected persons also
      with HIV/AIDS, 54
  number of infected persons, by
    nation, 18*t*

  in Papua New Guinea
    incidence, 59, 79*f*
    number of infected persons, 18*t*
  in Philippines
    incidence, 63, 79*f*
    number of infected persons, 18*t*
    percent of infected persons also
      with HIV/AIDS, 63
  as proxy for HIV/AIDS, 31
  in Thailand
    incidence, 55, 79*f*
    number of infected persons, 18*t*
    percent of infected persons also
      with HIV/AIDS, 55
  in Timor Leste
    number of infected persons, 18*t*
  treatment of, 18, 35
    planning for, 42–43
  in Vietnam
    incidence, 60, 79*f*
    number of infected persons, 18*t*
    percent of infected persons also
      with HIV/AIDS, 60
Tuvalu, number of HIV/AIDS-
  infected persons, 11

U

UNAIDS. *See* Joint United Nationals
  Program on HIV/AIDS
UNGASS. *See* United Nations Gen-
  eral Assembly Special Session on
  HIV/AIDS
UNICEF. *See* United Nations Chil-
  drens Fund
United Kingdom, anti-HIV/AIDS
  programs, 32–33
United Nations, anti-HIV/AIDS
  programs and, 5
United Nations Childrens Fund
  (UNICEF)
  anti-HIV/AIDS programs, 41
  Web site, 97
United Nations Development Pro-
  gramme (UNDP)
  anti-HIV/AIDS programs, 53, 55,
    56, 57, 60, 61, 62, 63
  Web site, 97

United Nations General Assembly
Special Session on HIV/AIDS
(UNGASS) [2001], 5, 19, 27
United Nations Office on Drugs and
Crime (UNODC), 41
United States, surveillance in, 41
UNODC. *See* United Nations Office
on Drugs and Crime
U.S. Agency for International Devel-
opment (USAID)
anti-HIV/AIDS programs, 23,
40–41, 41, 61, 63
Asian Epidemic Model
development of, 15–16, 76–77
predictions for Cambodia, 16
predictions for Thailand, 16, 21,
77, 88n
Web site, 97
U.S. Centers for Disease Control and
Prevention (CDC), 20, 21
U.S. Central Intelligence Agency
(CIA), 75
USAID. *See* U.S. Agency for Interna-
tional Development

V
Vietnam
antiretroviral patients, 60
blood supply safety in, 60
drug use, intravenous, 60, 67t
Global Fund funding, 60, 86t
GNI per capita, 12t, 60
incidence of HIV/AIDS, predicted
trends in, 76
mode of HIV transmission, 60
multidrug resistance in, 60
number of HIV/AIDS-infected
persons, 12t, 18t
population, 12t, 18t, 60
prevalence of HIV/AIDS, 12t, 14,
18t, 50f, 60, 67t
prevalence of SDIs, 76
response to HIV/AIDS, 27, 37, 40
funding of, 37, 60, 86t
sex workers
HIV/AIDS prevalence, 12t, 60, 69t
number and characteristics of, 69t

surveillance in, 31, 41
tuberculosis in
incidence, 60, 79f
number of infected persons, 18t
percent of infected persons also
with HIV/AIDS, 60
World Bank anti-HIV/AIDS
efforts in, 60

W
Women
in antenatal care clinics, HIV
prevalence
in Cambodia, 12t, 53
in China, 12t, 56
in Indonesia, 12t, 57
in Lao PDR, 13t, 61
in Malaysia, 12t, 58
in Mongolia, 13t, 62
in Myanmar, 12t, 54
in Papua New Guinea, 12t, 59
in Philippines, 13t, 63
in Thailand, 12t, 55
in Vietnam, 12t, 60
mother-child transmission, prevention of, 35
vulnerability to HIV/AIDS, 17, 33
World Bank
anti-HIV/AIDS efforts
in Cambodia, 53
in China, 56
efficacy of, 38–39
funding of, 4, 5, 23, 24, 37–38,
40, 45–46
in Indonesia, 57
lessons learned from, 39
in Malaysia, 58
monitoring of, 8, 38–39
in Papua New Guinea, 59
role in, 5–6, 9, 30, 39, 40, 41, 45,
46–47
in Thailand, 55
in Vietnam, 60
anti-HIV/AIDS strategy, 7–9, 41–47
analytic and advisory work in, 9, 45
funding in, 45–46

World Bank (*cont.*)
   anti-HIV/AIDS strategy, (*cont.*)
     policies, 41–45
     regional tools, 9, 46–47
   anti-tuberculosis efforts, 18
   and health spending accountability,
     36
   lending in EAP Region, 5, 9, 37, 46
   Web site, 97

World Bank Institute, 46–47
World Health Organization (WHO)
   and anti-HIV/AIDS programs, 5,
     23, 40, 41
   and health spending accountability,
     36
   3 by 5 initiative, 40
   on tuberculosis, 17, 18
   Web site, 97

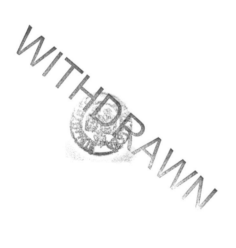